9.19

Start pg. 19, pg. 20 (brushes) pg. 21

9.29

A Guide to Beautiful Skin for Black Men and Women

By James A. Farabee

Illustrated by Culverson Blair

DOUBLEDAY & COMPANY, INC.
GARDEN CITY, NEW YORK
1983

Library of Congress Cataloging in Publication Data

Farabee, James A.
   A guide to beautiful skin for black men and
women.

   1. Skin—Care and hygiene.   2. Beauty,
Personal.   3. Blacks—Health and hygiene.
I. Title.
RL87.F37   616.5′05′08996073   AACR2
ISBN: 0-385-15512-3
Library of Congress Catalog Card Number: 79–8921

My parents . . . the champagne and the night I was
conceived . . . I've been effervescent ever since.

America where brilliance is commonplace . . .
I'm glad to have been born an American.

Acknowledgments

I EMBRACE this opportunity to say a fabulous thank-you, in order of appearance, to:

Ronald McGarrah—for lighting the direction.
Marie D. Brown—editor.
Rufus Still—patron of the art of just-in-time.
Janell Walden—for tailoring the order of events.
Dr. Richard J. Coburn—his brilliance epitomizes the glamour of his profession.
Dr. Lois E. Bradshaw—La Sparkle from center stage.
Culverson Blair—artist of fine lines.
Larry Naar—new beginnings, the best finish.
Christine Valmy—diva of American skin care.
Anthony Capibanico—caps and copies.
Michael Dash—the runner.
Robert Dockstader—for magic music.
Bravo and thanks to L. Law for makeup.
The chorus of models, actors, dancers—stars of tomorrow, for their faces and shapes: a special bravo for a job well done.
And to you—for turning the page to my innate beauty secrets.

Contents

Introduction

UNTIL RECENTLY dark-complexioned people in the United States had to depend almost entirely on products created primarily for the white skins of the Anglo-European-American majority in this country as the means of enhancing their black beauty. Rising incomes and the growing affirmation that now "black is beautiful" have created a new, growing market for cosmetics formulated exclusively for the dark skin. Some of the largest cosmetic houses are entering the field along with smaller, specialty houses. Yet their products aren't very likely by themselves to help the dark-skinned men and women who use them achieve their dreamed-of goal of an attractive complexion. In fact, many of these new products may be more a part of the problem than a part of the solution.

The reason is simple. Beauty is indeed more than skin deep. Complexion quality is the product of a varied and constantly changing array of influences, both internal and external, both emotional and physical, that affect our looks.

On the one hand, beauty emanates from the depths of one's mind and thoughts and, as such, is in a continual process of evolution. How we feel about ourselves has a profound influence on our appearance. On the other hand, the lifestyles we adopt to express our feelings about ourselves have a progressive and lasting physical effect on our complexions.

In today's world, for the active and affluent young man or woman, those lifestyles can be unbelievably demanding because we compress many different existences into a very short period. We move hourly, with ease, from harried executive to business traveler to active sportsperson to city sophisticate. This kind of ever-changing, fast-paced lifestyle exposes our skin to a varying array of environments and stresses which, with bewildering swiftness, have a debilitating effect on our skin.

Unless we take steps to preserve the youthful good looks and complexion quality that are everyone's heritage, all the foundation creams and rouges, toners, liners, and lipsticks on the new black cosmetic shelf that began as enhancements for youth's freshness will merely end up as camouflage for fading or faded beauty.

Only a rigorous and carefully designed beauty care system, begun as early as possible, centered on the skin and taking into account the many influences on its beauty, can offer hope for preserving and enhancing natural beauty for as long as possible.

Such a system has never existed for dark-skinned people. The techniques and regimens that did exist were evolved for people with lighter skins and with different lifestyles.

This problem has concerned me for a long time. As a result, I have made many visits—to "in" doctors in Manhattan's fashionable East Sixties and Seventies whose practice involves corrective beauty care as well as to instant beauty clinics and Europe's top spas. And I have studied with eminent cosmetologists and beauty experts, as well as with dermatologists and plastic surgeons.

Now, after ten years of study and research with beauty authorities in Europe, the United States, and Africa, I have developed a basic knowledge about the cosmetic care of dark skin. From this knowledge, I have formulated a beauty system of glorious secrets. I have utilized my system—my own approaches and techniques—in practice and teaching in my salon; and I have served as a referral service for those of my clients who needed specialized help beyond the salon. I have researched the causes and effects of most common beauty problems—acne, blackheads, blotches, dry skin, and so forth —as they appear in dark complexions. In short, I have a thorough knowledge of dark-skin problems and what must be done to maintain beauty in the black woman and black man.

It is now time for me to share this knowledge with you. In these pages I will show you a home skin care regimen that relies mainly on a few basic operations you can perform daily, using natural materials and inexpensive compounds available at your druggist's. This regimen can help you to create a personalized beauty care discipline tailored to your individual skin and its problem—or lack of problems. It includes variations to meet seasonal, geographic, or climatic changes; and the regimen is designed to evolve as you and your skin care needs evolve.

While these ideas are primarily for people who were born dark, many of them are also useful for people who choose to sun-darken their skins and who do not want to end up looking like a piece of leather at age forty. Further on, you will see my special strategies to counteract the premature onset of character lines, loss of skin elasticity, and other signs of aging.

The *Ananga Ranga*, a Hindu art-of-love epic written perhaps as early as the eleventh century, contains magic recipes for beautifying the skin and retarding its aging processes. There are no such magic potions in today's world, but it is my fond hope that by following the secrets set forth in this book, we may preserve ourselves a little longer and a little better, and in that sense be eternally beautiful.

J.A.F.

1

The Heritage
of Dark Skin

WE CAN NO LONGER accept the fact that dark skins should follow the accepted rules for Anglo-Saxon skin care. The dark complexion requires new moods, new feelings, and, above all else, new complexion standards from its own ancient beauty heritage for its Western way of life.

"I am black, but comely . . ." Thus spoke the central figure of the Song of Solomon in one of the most lyrical passages in the Old Testament and one of the most beautiful love poems of biblical culture. Its lyric speaks to the beauty of the human body, to the beauty of love, to the beauty of sex, to the beauty of life.

The poem is one of the wonderful traditions with which we of dark skin are graced, and it is no accident that its central figure, the bride, is black. Anthropology has it that far away in the mists of time the first humans appeared in Africa. From Africa they spread throughout the world—into Europe and into Asia—to form the various races of man. So my features are as much Ethiopian/Egyptian/East Indian as they are American/Baltimore, Maryland. According to anthropological theory, as migration continued into colder climates, those with lighter skins that could absorb the sun's health-giving rays and who therefore stood a better chance of survival continued their migration, thus seasoning the complexions of the world, while those with darker ones returned to Africa. Therefore, as the story goes, over millions of years of migration, all the shades of skin came about.

Yet this may be only a fascinating myth since, as we shall see later in this chapter, the little cells that make skin color brown or black are just as numerous in white skins—they simply produce much less color in light skins.

But the mystique of dark skin reaches far beyond the confines of Africa. Dark skin—smooth, supple, velvety to the touch, sensuous in every way—is central to the romance of the tropics and appreciation of its vitality and comeliness has bred hordes of lighter-skinned sun worshipers in colder climates who yearn for and crowd to the places that offer them a touch of this mystique.

By caravans and conquest, African beauty practices have influenced the world and gold, ivory, spices, and slaves were brought from African empires. Arrival of African slaves in the New World established African beauty lore farther abroad and made way for the Afro-Caribbean cultures and the variations in complexion we know so well today.

African beauty practices survived Europe's Dark Ages into the Renaissance and after. Beauties such as Marie Antoinette adapted African beauty formulas and put them in bottles and jars. Thus many European cosmetic preparations traced their origins to Africa.

To this very day, in every cosmetic invention for even the fairest blond complexion there lies a dark drop of beauty magic that has its origin in the melting of Mount Kilimanjaro's snows.

This, then, is the legacy of our dark skin, the heritage of our beauty secrets. To learn how to tap this legacy and these secrets, to best meet your own beauty needs, you will first need to know about your skin and how it functions.

YOUR SKIN: A CRESCENDO IN HUE

Skin holds no mystery. It simply has a life of its own and will react to that life when you least think about it. It pops out in rashes, gets a pimple here or there, is alternately dull, clammy, or flaky without even so much as a warning. If you understand that your skin has life and how your skin's life relates to the rest of you, then your skin will hold no mystery.

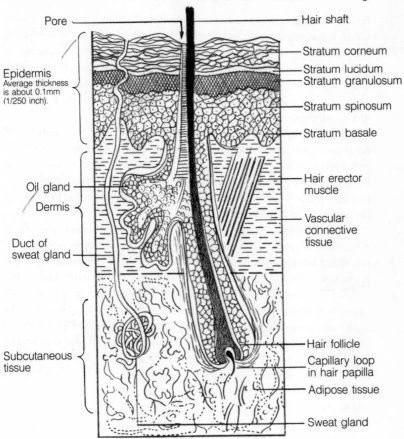

Pore — Hair shaft

Epidermis
Average thickness
is about 0.1mm
(1/250 inch).

Stratum corneum
Stratum lucidum
Stratum granulosum
Stratum spinosum
Stratum basale

Oil gland
Dermis

Hair erector
muscle

Vascular
connective
tissue

Duct of
sweat gland

Subcutaneous
tissue

Hair follicle
Capillary loop
in hair papilla
Adipose tissue

Sweat gland

Layers of skin.

When people bother to think of their skin at all, many think of it as a kind of marvelous wrapper for their bodies, like a glorious mink coat. Stand before a mirror and look at it. If it isn't sleek, smooth, and oh, so soft to the touch, then you can make it so, because it is the nature of the skin to respond with surprising speed to tender loving care.

For the skin is far more than a wrapper for your body. It is a wonderfully complicated vital organ of protection, sense, elimination, and regulation. As a protector, the wrapper guards against infection and keeps out unwanted dirt and other foreign elements, while allowing life-sustaining vital body fluids in. It also protects sensitive inner tissues from the harmful effects of the environment. As a sense organ, as all lovers well know, it responds to gentle touch, to mood, to music, and to pressure, to heat and to cold. The wrapper helps in the elimination of the body's waste materials and in the regulation of body temperature.

Most beautiful people appreciate their skin as a fine-textured natural fabric. On the average, this fabric is only about 2.5 millimeters thick, though its thickness varies. The palms of the hands, soles of the feet, and other areas of friction tend to be thicker, while the eyelids, inner elbows, and in some human groups the lips tend to be thinner.

If you could shed your skin to weigh it, it would represent about 5 percent of your total body weight if you are neither too fat nor too thin. Man or woman, fat or thin, your skin is by far your largest organ.

Like the rest of your body, your skin comprises many invisibly small building blocks of living matter called "cells." Although the many kinds of cells that we will explore are organized in a myriad of ways, basically you need only be concerned with the two layers, the epidermis and dermis, which for the romance of it we will call the "allegro" and the "adagio." The allegro's function is primarily to form and maintain the body's flexible, waterproof outer layer, while the adagio performs all the other functions.

Both the allegro and adagio layers have several layers of their own, each displaying its own character and function. To understand how the various treatments in this book work, you need to know a few facts about many of these layers.

As we all know, when a burn or scrape removes the top layer of skin, exposing the quick, or red underlying tissue, it is extremely painful. The area is agonizingly sensitive to touch, to the application of "soothing" ointments, and even to a breath. (Cold water and an application of natural talc may be helpful.) The area oozes clear body fluids or bleeds, will always form a dry, rigid scab, and may even become infected. This is clear evidence that inner tissues cannot withstand the outside world and are reliant for their safe functioning on the outer skin.

So what is this miracle that creates a surface both functional and beautiful and is able to withstand environmental assaults while able to respond with exquisite feeling to a lover's touch?

YOUR ALLEGRO—THE OUTER SKIN, OR EPIDERMIS

The secret lies in the epidermis, which consists of many cell layers in various stages of growth and maturation, from the innermost fragile water-fat cells to the outermost tough waterproof cells made mostly of the protein keratin. In addition to being in your skin, keratin is found in your hair and nails—in animals, in hooves and horns!

The innermost layer of cells is in constant rhythm and harmony, dividing and multiplying through three stages of transformation as they move outward to become the outermost layer of keratin-filled cells that flake away constantly to make room for new layers in this continuum of skin growth.

Each newborn, innermost cell is cylindrical in shape, contains a nucleus that governs the cell's function, and is fat with moisture. In its first transformation it grows rounder, then begins to flatten as it loses moisture. At this same flattening stage it begins to form particles that will contribute to its ultimate substance, keratin; many of the cells display tiny projecting fibers that grip each other to form interlocking tissue. In its final stage of transformation, the cell nucleus, whose governing job is done, has disappeared; the cell is now almost all keratin and contains very little moisture, one of the billions of tiny overlapping cells that form the outermost layer of your skin.

This constant magical transformation cycle of the cell from its formation to its emergence as outer layer takes approximately twenty-seven days.

Many internal and external forces acting on your skin can interfere dramatically with the schedule for this skin growth process. Sunburn can prematurely damage still-living cells, speeding up and changing the separation of outer layers in what we know as "peeling." Continuous mild friction or pressure can cause the cells to hang on longer than normal, thus forming thickened calluses on your skin. Hard rubbing, especially of light- or thin-textured skin, can result in a complete separation of the allegro and adagio layers to form a protective pad of healing fluid—a blister—over the injured area.

Chemical and electrical signals carried to the skin through the vascular and nervous systems can sometimes accelerate the skin growth process too rapidly and cause problems. One is the red flakiness seen in psoriasis, a condition resulting from the growth process occurring ten times faster than normal. (Saltwater compresses may reduce the redness.) Another such problem is dandruff, resulting from too much shedding too soon of the outer cell layer of the scalp. (Pine tar shampoo used regularly is helpful in controlling dandruff.)

The ends of the pain- and heat-sensing nerves and the bottom layers of the allegro are given their start in life and nurtured by blood vessels in the second, inner layer of the skin, the adagio, or dermis. The nourishment passes from the adagio's tiny, tiny vessels to the allegro through an infinitely thin tissue layer called stratum basale or basement membrane.

THE IMPORTANT ADAGIO

Although it is thought that many common skin problems come from interference in the normal process of allegro growth and shedding, most other problems are associated with pores, the glandular and follicular openings in the adagio and the allegro.

If you think the structure and function of the allegro seem somewhat complicated, believe me they are sheer simplicity when compared to the adagio, which is packed with both blood and lymph vessels, nerves, sweat glands, oil glands, hair follicles, tiny muscles called "arrectores pilorum" (hair erector muscles), and a variety of other components, some whose function is only beginning to be understood and doubtless others yet to be identified and named!

Holding together this seeming plethora of adagio components is a dense network of connective tissue, consisting primarily of collagen and elastin fibers. These fibers give the skin its suppleness and tone, so it is important that any moisturizer you use have a collagen content. These components can be damaged or destroyed by too much sunlight taken for too long periods of time. Their breakdown through improper sunning can lead, mostly in light and white skins, to premature aging of your skin and sometimes to skin cancer.

In the deepest adagio layer are found the fat cells. These cells vary in number and size according to sex, nutrition, and location in the body. And, they contribute those delectable curves men do so love in women!

Finally, special pigment cells that manufacture brown or black pigment, or melanin, that determines your skin color begin in the adagio, then extend through the basement membrane to the allegro.

An excellent illustration of your skin's importance to your whole system is the fact that at any one time your skin contains one third of the body's circulating blood.

THE FIRST BREW: PERSPIRATION

Have you ever wondered why you can sweat heavily all over your body, yet produce a strong smell only under your arms and in other closed places? It's because you have two kinds of sweat glands— eccrine and apocrine—which empty out of your pores.

Your approximately 2 million ordinary eccrine sweat glands secrete a colorless, odorless fluid through your pores in response to heat to help cool the body by evaporation. This fluid, which is water with traces of salts, lactate, and urea, is also released in response to stress. The eccrine glands are freely distributed over virtually every hairless skin area of your body, thickest on your soles and palms and nonexistent only on the very tip of the male sexual organ.

The other sweat glands, the apocrine glands, are not nearly so numerous and are connected to hair follicles, primarily in the underarm, genital, and anal areas. In response to exertion, stress, or lovemaking, the apocrine glands secrete through your pores a thick, slightly milky substance which is odorless when it is first secreted. External and airborne bacteria attack and break down these secretions to produce that old devil body odor!

But the human senses are discriminating when it comes to body odor. Some body odor we find offensive and attempt to ameliorate or cover up our own with deodorants, antiperspirants, and fragrances. Yet other body odor we find erotic. Some lovemakers say there is no scent so enticingly powerful as the one they get with a little "hard exercise" just after a shower. This scent, unfortunately, will never be bottled.

Some scientists now believe that the odors resulting from apocrine gland secretions carry not only sexual messages but psychological messages as well that affect menstrual cycles and other subtle body processes.

Some of your pores perform double or even triple duty. As we have seen, there are apocrine sweat glands with hair follicles connected to some pores, eccrine sweat glands connected to others. And now we add oil glands to the others. Their scientific name, sebaceous glands, is derived from their secretion, sebum. For simplicity, however, let's just use "oil glands" and "oil."

Keeping your pores open and functioning is a major objective of our skin care regime. Clogged oil glands are the cause of blackheads, whiteheads, acne, and other problems, while clogged or overloaded sweat glands can cause painful and troublesome blistering or rashes.

A hair follicle opening has another fascinating property: It will close up to become a goose bump in response to cold, fear, or anger. This is caused by that tiny muscle, arrector pili, which is attached to the follicle. When it tightens, it also makes the hair stand upright.

You may also wonder why your skin is oily in areas where there seem to be no hairs—your nose and forehead, for example—or why you can have goose bumps on your arms and back. The answer is that there are hairs on these areas but they are so fine as to be almost invisible. In fact, the vast majority of your hair follicles do not grow "real" hair of the kind you find on your head or chin. But they have all the other properties, and that's why you can get an acne pimple almost anyplace. It is also why good grooming must include the chest and back as well as the face.

THE PLEASING TONE . . . THE RIGHT COLORING

Human skin color is determined largely by a substance called "melanin," the pigment that gives dark-skinned people their brown or black color and enables light-skinned people to get suntans. It is produced by pigment cells that are located, as mentioned before, in the basement membrane between the adagio and the allegro. Also as mentioned earlier, the number of pigment cells is about the same for every race, and there is no need in nature to change a good pattern. What does determine, for the most part, the variations in black, brown, red, yellow, and white skin colors is the type and the way the pigment cells are distributed.

Two other substances affect skin color to a marked degree—carotene and hemoglobin. Carotene, the second pigment, is in fatty epidermal cells and gives them a yellow color. Incidentally, it is the same substance that gives carrots and other yellow vegetables their color. So, for those needing yellow to balance skin tone, I suggest eating lots of carrots, as they actually give your skin a yellow tint. Plan your intake to match your mood—munch on a fresh carrot, have some cool fresh carrot juice, or brew a raw carrot in your morning tea or drip its juice into your coffee.

Hemoglobin, which is an iron compound, is the substance in your blood that carries oxygen from your lungs to all your cells and gives the blood its red color. Since one third of your blood at any one time is circulating through the skin, the amount and redness of the blood will impart pinkish or reddish tones to your skin.

All human skin remaining in the same environments for millennia develop the coloring necessary for survival. Your skin is not only a marvelously complex organism, but also a miraculously responsive one which reacts in different ways to environmental changes—to the external forces of sun, wind, heat and cold, moisture and dryness.

Most of the skin's reactions are normal—that is, they are the skin's proper responses to the forces that act upon it. My skin care program is intended to help the skin deal effectively and positively with these reactions, foster the natural beauty of the skin, to influence it in such a way as to bring about long-lasting protective results. Since in today's world it is impossible simply to change one's environment to suit one's beauty needs, my program is designed to help your skin find and use its own beauty secrets in whatever environment you are. Corrective measures, where they are possible, are a last resort in my skin care program.

EXTERNAL FORCES THAT AFFECT YOUR SKIN

The Sun—Mother Goddess

There are perhaps no more ancient religious mysteries than those having to do with the power of the sun. Ancient peoples throughout the world worshiped the sun as Mother Goddess, the source of life, and recognized clearly its healing powers. In the Christian era in Europe, after sun worship disappeared, it was centuries before people learned the therapeutic values of the sun. Finally, in the late nineteenth century, history records its rediscovery—to kill bacteria and in the prevention and/or cure of various diseases and disorders such as rickets, tuberculosis, acne, eczema, and psoriasis.

Yet, as we all know, the heat rays of our Mother Protector the sun can be damaging to the skin as well as beneficial. Especially for light-skinned people, but for dark-skinned people as well, too lengthy exposure to too strong sunrays can induce negative skin effects ranging from dryness to painful and serious burns to premature aging!

Since so large a part of today's "good life" takes place out of doors in the sunlight, it is essential that you understand how the sun affects your skin and how you can protect your skin from its harm while gloriously reaping its benefits.

It is not the sun's light or heat that cause sunburn or kill bacteria. It is the sun's invisible ultraviolet rays, which cannot be felt but which can penetrate the clouds to sunburn you even on a day when the sky is overcast. These ultraviolet rays are similar to the "black lights" in discos, which show off what's on you and make things glow fluorescently in the dark. There are some things ultraviolet rays can't penetrate however—ordinary windowglass and cloth other than very, very sheer material.

Ultraviolet rays cannot penetrate a good sunscreen preparation. And, a silk cloth dyed with vegetable coloring can be helpful if you cannot be out in the sun without getting painfully burned.

That many white-skinned persons are sun worshipers longing for that beautiful bronzed look is attested to by the throngs of people on the beaches in summer. Few seem concerned that, though skin experts are divided on the subject, most European skin specialists say that the benefits probably aren't worth what you have to pay for the bronzing.

How to use sunlight for cosmetic and therapeutic purposes will be discussed in detail in Chapter 4, "Treatments Just for You."

Wind

The wind alone, or in combination with the sun, is a force that can have a powerful negative effect on your skin. Even the gentlest breeze can lull you into a feeling of security long enough for you not to realize that you are getting a severe sunburn. A brisk breeze when the humidity is low can dry out your skin very quickly, especially in cold weather. For this reason, you should oil your complexion during winter months.

Windburn, more noticeable in light-skinned people, characterized by irritated redness and dry flaking or scaling, is caused by dehydration. Windburn is common among skiers, who may lessen or eliminate the effect of wind by drinking more liquids and massaging exposed skin with a light corn oil.

Chapping is a more severe condition, characterized by loss of most of the moisture and flexibility of the allegro, resulting in brittle, cracked skin that may even cause bleeding, particularly on the lips. If you skin gets chapped, you can be sure you have not moisturized it adequately.

Air and Water

Dry air can be a constant enemy of your skin's moisture balance, be it the result of indoor winter heat, outdoor cold, or desert conditions. And, you must protect yourself from these drynesses. Corrective skin treatments are the same, no matter what the dry air results from. If your skin becomes dry from any dry air, apply water and oil in separate applications.

Water, too, can be your skin's enemy, but particularly when some chemicals or other substances have been added to it. And because of air pollution we bathe often—this may mean too much contact with water, which causes the skin to lose its natural ability to hold moisture.

For the pool swimmer extra precaution is necessary to prevent damage to skin from too much "treated" water. For this I recommend a saltwater spray after pool swimming.

Your skin gives you an excellent warning that you've been in any water too long when it begins to wrinkle. Even too many baths at home and failure to dry the skin totally can contribute to skin dryness.

Heat and Cold

I would suggest that you use lukewarm water for all home washing and bathing since both heat and cold extremes decrease body moisture and tend to have a drying effect on your skin.

Air heat, particularly dry heat, puts the sweat glands to work releasing fluids to cool your body. If the pores that carry the fluid are blocked or if too much sweat is produced for the ducts to carry, a number of unpleasant and uncomfortable skin textures such as itching and chapping can ensue.

Moist air heat, however, can be very helpful as it stimulates the skin gently without drying it; encourages the pores to open and, if they happen to be clogged, it unclogs them; and softens the shedding allegro. This is why saunas are so beneficial to your skin and make you feel so good.

The body scent caused by the heating of the skin is not always found offensive—in fact, it can bring people together. Legend has it that amour often happened at court after dancing, and that in Eastern courts, dancing girls were allegedly more wanted after they performed, thanks to the scent of their heated skin from the crushed osmunda plant rubbed on their bodies beforehand. While you don't have to dance for your lover (you can if you want to, of course), put a flowery fragrance on your body before your lovemaking begins and see what beauty happens!

On the other hand, heat can aggravate the problems of people who have skin problems associated with enlarged surface blood vessels.

When you are cold, your surface blood vessels get smaller, causing the blood to remain deeper in your body to keep you warm, as if you were drawing your body up inside a cuddly warm fur coat.

Your sweat glands produce less fluids and your pores become closed-up goose bumps. I suggest an oil massage before any outdoor activity in very cold weather to help keep your skin soft and elastic.

Prolonged exposure to freezing temperatures can result in mild-to-severe cosmetic and health damage as well as considerable discomfort. Although most of us are too savvy these days to let so foolish a thing happen, it's good to remind ourselves of the dangers of extreme cold. ✓

Chilblains, a mild degree of frostbite affecting toes, fingers, and ears, can cause recurrent itching and swelling and can result in dark skin areas that may or may not go away. In more severe frostbite, your skin and underlying tissues actually freeze, which can result in scarring and tissue loss. In the excitement of outdoor activities, it is easy for you to ignore warning symptoms of frostbite such as tingling and numbness; but don't—ignoring numbness is nothing but dumbness! Warming or thawing of frostbitten areas should be gradual and started before going into the warmth of indoors. Warm mint tea with lime, hot chocolate, or a wonderful Danish concoction of warm red wine, almonds, nutmeg, and brandy are all good for a gradual warming.

Dust and Air Pollutants

Your skin's natural oils and moisture form an ideal trap for any dust, smoke, or other airborne substances present in your daily environment. These substances may be mildly irritating in themselves, so you must take steps to protect your skin from them. If these pollutants cannot be warded off, then together with accumulation of secretions and dead epidermal cells, they should be carefully cleansed from the skin to keep it healthy. A dark skin may produce more oil and moisture than a white one even if the accumulation doesn't show. You must remove it all in order to prevent irritation and clogging of your pores.

Cosmetic Irritants

I feel that most makeup is put on to cover up the effects of poor skin care, to create another complexion, and that most of us would be better off and more beautiful if we relied on the natural beauty of our own healthy skins rather than on attempts to improve nature by painting our faces!

In ancient Africa, makeup was put on as protection from danger, to color oneself to blend in with the jungle. Today makeup is used to make you stand out, for attractiveness, and subtle highlighting or accents can bring out the best in your face. But always remember, nothing takes the place of good skin care!

A complexion gained from makeup will wear out if you don't know how to apply it. Makeup may clog your pores and be irritating as well, since colors and coatings, foundations, rouges, liners, and such have much the same effect on your skin as dust and pollution. Again, regular basic skin care is a must for a beautiful you!

Friction

The causes of calluses and blisters have been dealt with already, so let's talk a little about friction.

A frequent result of friction in our everyday lives is skin discoloration from elastics or binding clothing on our bodies. Simply rubbing skin regularly against any rough texture can produce such discoloration, in fact. Especially in dark-skinned people, darkening of the skin may result. Take a look at your body. Almost everyone experiences some darkening from friction at the elbows, knees, and buttocks.

Or you may find yourself from time to time with friction scrapes from sliding falls on wooden floors when you're playing or doing exercises.

Regardless of the cause, you should always treat friction scrapes and discolorations first with a carbolated petroleum jelly and cool-water rinse. Soaking in Epsom salts promotes healing.

INTERNAL INFLUENCES

Your Diet

An apple from a tree is, like a banana, secret and magical food for the gods. However, there is no one magic beauty food that can give you magnificent skin, although your skin, like the rest of your body, will respond to your diet either positively or negatively. You are, as they say, what you eat.

When you do not get enough of the necessary nutrients, either through food alone or food in combination with supplements, your skin is frequently one of the first parts of your body to show signs of deficiency. You can see and feel the difference if you know your skin well. There will be a loss of skin tone; this happens periodically to almost everyone and calls for remedial action.

Loss of skin tone and texture, with slackening and wrinkling of skin, as well as hair loss, may indicate a protein deficiency. Dry scaly skin may indicate insufficient intake of essential fatty acids.

Certain foods may cause skin problems, for some people. But some foods that have been accused of causing problems probably do not. I no longer think, for instance, that the amount of fat in your diet has much to do with the oiliness of your skin. On the other hand, I do believe that certain chemicals and hormones used in crop and livestock production can affect your skin's oiliness. Other foods, not surprisingly, can make your skin ultralovely. Among these are lime juice, sweet potatoes, carrots, and celery, as well as mint and garlic.

Beware of crash diets and excessive thinness. They're just not good for your skin.

Your General State of Health

Food, entertainment, sex . . . the three real reasons for which many find themselves on earth! And if you are to enjoy them fully, your body's overall condition must be excellent. And if it is, your skin will show it glowingly.

Your skin often reflects health problems—and can be a signal to you to seek medical care. For example, yellowish or gray-green skin color reflects impaired liver function, which may be due to too much alcohol, infection, or a combination of the two.

You will certainly not have a glowing skin or a magnificent complexion if your body's overall condition is bad.

Storm and Stress

Many of your emotional experiences affect your skin. If you worry too much, you may get a pimple, or many pimples, because the worrying increases production of hormones, which over-stimulates the oil glands, which overworks and clogs the pores—and there comes a pimple.

Long-continued stress can dilate your blood vessels, sensitize your nerve endings, cause excessive sweating, and, in short, just plain totally disrupt your skin's normal balance. The best treatment for stress is to prevent it . . . to remember not to be a part of it. It is no longer a part of a black's successful step forward.

Stress can also cause you to drink too much, pop too many pills, neglect your diet, and end up damaging your overall health as well as your skin. If you let this happen, you are foolish, and it is time for you to change your attitude!

You must treat yourself well! Eat well. Exercise. Get enough rest. Meditate. Pamper yourself. Make love. Slow down and enjoy life. And always, ritually follow your skin care program!

A seer once told a group, "Embarrassment felt in our mind is instantly reflected on our skin." Don't let embarrassing reflections happen to you. Let me help your wonderful beauty emerge, by letting you in on the beauty secrets of a historical people and leading you to discover your very own.

2

Your Skin Care Apothecary

BOTH the pharmacy counter and the grocery shelf offer you many substances of high quality that do all the things for your skin expensive cosmetic-counter products do, but at a much lower cost. In fact, the corner drugstore has sparked many beauties!

Your pharmacist can be a valuable source of help and advice about preparations for your skin. Often he can make up simple compounds that are better than their equivalent "brand" versions. He will also probably know the latest patent preparations for specific problems.

A budget skin care apothecary of your own need not sacrifice either quality or luxury. Economics is a matter of taste . . . but your own apothecary just leaves you more money for greater luxury where it really counts! For example, say your pharmacist compounds a moisturizer for five dollars that would cost you twelve to fifteen dollars at the cosmetic counter. That leaves you over ten dollars to spend on some tremendous soap or exotic bath oil. Or, how about a good bottle of wine to have today while you are pampering your entire body from head to toe?

By using a careful selection of simple drugstore materials and some wholesome ingredients from grocery and health food stores, you can make cosmetic preparations yourself that are more luxurious than any you can buy and at a fraction of the cost.

The Beauty Chef's homemade cosmetic preparations have three great advantages over ones you buy:

- *Your products will not contain unnecessary stabilizers and preservatives that have nothing to do with your skin's condition.* These ingredients are necessary in commercial preparations, however, to increase their shelf life, to maintain their quality during shipment, and to improve the way they look.
- *You can tailor your preparations to your own skin's needs.* Unlike a commerical product, which must suit many different kinds of skin, your preparation is just for you. You know all its ingredients, so you can avoid substances that irritate or cause an allergic reaction in your skin.
- *Yours is a very special total beauty-making treatment.* You have the makings of your very own beauty secrets . . . above all, the special beauty treatment just for you.

Remember, in using any preparation mentioned in this book, or, in making up cosmetics from the recipes, THERE IS NO COSMETIC PREPARATION THAT CAN BE GUARANTEED TO BE ABSOLUTELY SAFE FOR EVERYONE UNDER ALL CONDITIONS OF USE.

It is very easy for you to test any ingredient or cosmetic preparation on your skin for possible sensitivity—and it is very important that you always test anything new that you use:

- Apply the substance to a small area on the inside of your forearm.
- Cover it with an adhesive bandage.
- Leave it alone for twenty-four hours.
- If there is a reaction—rashes, redness, etc.—avoid the substance.

To continue to be safe, always take care to follow directions given on the product exactly and watch closely for any reaction the first few times you use a preparation. If there *is* a reaction, stop using the substance immediately. If the reaction is severe, see your doctor.

TOOLS OF YOUR TRADE
—BASIC BEAUTIES HAVE EVERYTHING

Whatever substances and preparations you finally choose for your skin care apothecary, there is a basic assortment of tools and accessories you will need for your beauty treatment. And I suggest that you get these first, since nothing is more frustrating than to have your lovely array of beauty products all ready but your day of pampering come to naught for want of a cotton square!

Since there are so few of these items and they are so important to your beauty and well-being, I think you should spare no expense to make your collection the best you can possibly get. Note I said "collection," meaning it is built up over time. If you must begin with economy-quality items, do. But then move up to luxury, item by item, as you can. Remember that the money you save by making your own cosmetic preparations more than justifies splurging on your paraphernalia!

Here are my suggestions for your basic equipment:

For your preparations

Small mortar and pestle (heavy glass or marble); absolutely essential for grinding ingredients.

Blender (your kitchen one is fine); essential for your smooth masks and creams.

Glass bottles (at least a dozen, 4 to 6 ounces); for storing just the right amount of your liquids. (MORE)

Jars (at least a dozen glass ones, not over 4 ounces); for storing your creamy preparations. (more)

Atomizer (1 or 2 beautiful glass ones); for spraying on your astringent and freshener.

Steamer; for preparing vegetable washes.

For your applications

• Two dozen thin white cotton washcloths
• Gauze squares
• Cotton squares
• Cotton swabs

For your treatments and care

Tweezers (3 pairs); 1 with square tips, 1 with pointed tips, 1 with angled tips.

Scissors (2 pairs); 1 with pointed tips, 1 with blunted tips.

Metal dishpan (1); for footbaths—make it large enough for you to be able to stand in comfortably—metal stays warm longer.

Loofahs (3); for your many moods—1 with a glove, 1 square and flat, 1 round, big, and natural.

Pumice; for elbows, knees, and heels.

Safety razor (1 adjustable, with double-edged blade).

Feather body duster; for dusting on your scented talc, great for a tingling, sensual feeling.

Complexion and body brushes (some firm, some soft); fine brushes for face, neck, arms, elbows, knees, back, and feet.

About brushes . . . find the finest ones in special corners of beauty counters, drugstores, cosmetic shops, and natural food stores. They may be made of animal hair or vegetable fiber, but not synthetic fiber. No matter what your skin tone—jet black, brown-black, chestnut, copper, bronze, or whatever—you can literally sweep away any nasty undertones (underlying color that modifies your skin tone) that surface by brushing the skin. The tension of brushing accomplishes this. Brushing also stimulates circulation and cleanses deep down. ✓

YOUR OWN MINI-APOTHECARY

Your bathroom (which we'll get around to later) is your arsenal and your mini-apothecary of skin care. It contains the ammunition you'll need in your campaign to maintain your good looks and to offset the ill effects on your skin of air pollution, age, too much sun, inadequate care, and high living.

With the ingredients listed here (and a few more from your kitchen) and by following my recipes and treatments, you will be able to select just the ones best suited to you.

Once you have done that, you will have a relatively simple array of marvelous beauty secrets that are completely you and you alone —not anyone else and certainly not the average Joe or Josephine. Your cosmetics will be adaptable to travel in different climates, to changes of the seasons, and to the natural changes in your own skin.

YOUR BASICS

In all the profusion of names and compounds, there are only six basic kinds of skin care products:

• Cleansers

• Astringents
• Toners
• Masks
• Emollients

You generally use them in your skin care regimen in the order they are listed here. And you should know about each of them, so you can use them intelligently and for maximum beauty.

On the principle that simplicity is best, select one of each category that does its own particular job as well as it can be done. And don't expect one product to do two things—don't expect a soap to be a moisturizer or an astringent to be a toner.

Cleansers—Soaps, Creams, Lotions

In the pioneer and plantation days, our ancestors made their own soap out of animal fats and lye from wood ashes boiled in caldrons. Fortunately, those days are over. Today, soap manufacturing is an exact science, and since commercial soap is made with a wide range of properties, it is one of the few products that I recommend you buy right off the shelf.

Cosmetic soap manufacturers customarily make three general types of soaps:

• One for dry skin.
• One for oily skin.
• One for normal skin.

When you know your skin type (Chapter 3 will tell you how to find out), try several different brands of the soap suitable for your particular skin type to discover the very best one for you. Some soaps have scents, colorings, deodorants, or preservatives which you may not like or which may irritate your skin. So choose carefully.

Other skin cleansers are in the form of creams and lotions, which simply means they have more liquid in them than soaps.

No matter what their form, cleansers have the same functions: They dissolve and loosen the oil, fat, and dried sweat residue your pores secrete; they dissolve and loosen the flakes of epidermis you shed.

Astringents—Fresheners, Light Lotions

Astringents are used as stimulants and bracers for your skin. They close the pores, increase circulation, and tingle the nerve ends. They have antiseptic properties as well, which is why they cause open cuts to sting.

Most astringents have a degreasing effect. It is important to consider your skin type in selecting an astringent. If you have oily skin, choose one with a degreaser; if you have dry skin, choose one that is not a degreaser.

Rubbing alcohol is the most widely used skin astringent. (Caution: Do not take internally.) Other good astringents are citrus juices and acetone (never used full strength).

Toners—Liquids, Lotions

Dark-skinned people frequently have variations in skin color from one area of the face to another. Some of these are very subtle, others quite marked. They may be caused by variations in the underlying pigment, by local skin conditions, or by exposure to weather and climate. They may be quite flattering or they may be distracting and negative in their effect on your looks.

Toners are designed to even out skin color, change it subtly to flatter you even more, and create a balance in the skin itself that will be conducive to more even texture and tone. The most commonly used toners are witch hazel and citrus juices.

Masks

Masks are coatings applied to your face which dry and work on your skin for a period of time from about five minutes to a half hour or more.

Masks vary in their methods of application. Some must be put on heavily so that a "drawing" or feeding action can take place. Others are actually so light and transparent that you might put them on and then go out and do your grocery shopping or pick up the laundry without having to worry about your looks.

The group of masks designed to draw the skin remove unwanted oils and firm the underlying tissues. These are the familiar "mudpack" masks made from various earths, with the addition of other good things to help your skin. If you watch such a mask carefully as it dries on your face, you will see that some areas of the mask dry more slowly than others. These areas reveal the location of underlying skin that may be secreting too much oil and indicate where you should apply special strategies to balance your skin.

Other masks are designed to feed and moisturize your skin while they do their firming work. Some wonderful avocado-egg mixtures come to mind, as do a variety of cereal masks made from very fine flours full of vitamins and nourishing oils.

The action of your mask will vary according to the fluid you use to moisten the main ingredient, so that masks can be astringent, healing, and so forth. In fact, the combinations are almost endless. A few recipes I consider best are given later in the chapter.

Emollients—Moisturizers, Creams, Softeners

Emollients are compounds that keep your skin soft, supple, and velvety smooth. They are a mixture of water and oil or wax, the water to actually soften and the oil or wax to form a film that prevents the water from evaporating too soon.

The most familiar and commonly used emollient is cold cream, a wonderful invention of the Greek medical genius Galen, the court physician to the Roman emperor Marcus Aurelius (A.D. 121–180). He mixed olive oil, beeswax, and water with rose petals, to form a smooth, perfumed cream. Galen chose his ingredients well, for modern science has discovered that the composition of one of the substances formed in our skin's outer layer is very much like beeswax.

Some emollients contain extra ingredients that are helpful to your skin for other reasons. Collagen, for example, is an extract of protein that may be one of the ingredients of a more expensive emollient. Since collagen is one of the two chief building blocks of your dermis, its application externally is thought to be helpful in retaining the suppleness and softness of the dermis. Vitamins are also often found in emollients, especially vitamin E, which is supposed to help smooth wrinkles and nourish the skin. Urea, a chemical with an affinity for water, is often used to improve the moisture-retaining properties of less greasy emollients.

You should choose your cleanser, astringent, toner, mask, and emollient to suit the varying conditions that affect your skin and, of course, to suit the condition of your skin itself at any given time. A rare and lucky individual is the one who can use the same set of preparations the year round, regardless of the season, the climate, and the air quality. How to vary your choices of skin treatment preparations to suit these varying conditions will be covered in the next chapter.

FIFTY-THREE SUBSTANCES FOR YOUR APOTHECARY SHELF
(FOR EXTERNAL USE)

Oils
  Almond oil
  Camphor oil
  Garlic oil
  Oil of wintergreen
  Olive oil
  Vegetable oils

Herbs
  Chamomile
  Comfrey
  Ginseng
  Rosemary
  Sage

Cereals
  Barley meal
  Buckwheat meal
  Oatmeal

Earths
  Fuller's earth
  Kaolin

Spices
  Ginger
  Nutmeg

Astringents and Antiseptics
  Alcohol (rubbing)
  Alum (powder)
  Aluminum acetate (solution)
  Hydrogen peroxide (solution)
  Iodine (solution)
  Salt (Sodium chloride)
  Sodium perborate (solution)
  Spirits of camphor

Cleansers and Soothing Agents
  Bath salts
  Bicarbonate of soda (powder)
  Borax (crystals)
  Cold cream
  Milk of magnesia
  Vinegar (cider or wine)
  Zinc oxide (ointment)

Moisturizers
  Cocoa butter
  Glycerin

Powders
  Cornsilk powder
  Cornstarch
  Talc

Waters
  Fruit waters
  Orange-flower water

Rose water
Vegetable waters
Witch hazel

Lubricants
Mineral oil
Petroleum jelly
Texturized lard

Miscellaneous
Alkanet root
Aloe gel
Effervescents
Epsom salts
Medicated ointments
PABA cream
Paraffin wax

WHERE TO GET YOUR APOTHECARY SUBSTANCES

Drugstore
Alcohol
Aluminum acetate
Boric acid
Borax
Cocoa butter
Cornsilk powder
Effervescents
Fuller's earth
Glycerin
Hydrogen peroxide
Iodine solution
Kaolin
Milk of magnesia
Mineral oil
Petroleum jelly
Rose water
Sodium perborate
Spirits of camphor
Talc
Witch hazel
Zinc oxide

Supermarket
Alum

Bicarbonate of soda
Cornstarch
Fruit (for waters)
Ginger
Nutmeg
Oatmeal
Olive oil
Rosemary
Sage
Salt
Texturized lard
Vegetables (for waters)
Vinegar
Vegetable oils

Natural Food Stores
Alkanet root
Almond oil
Barley meal
Buckwheat meal
Chamomile
Comfrey
Ginseng
Orange-flower water

Oils

ALMOND OIL: A fragrant, bland and soothing oil used in creams. It can be used in a mask and for facial scrubs. Also used in soap.

OLIVE OIL: Probably the first oil used in cosmetics. Use only the finest and lightest—it penetrates the skin well. Used in the finest castile soap.

VEGETABLE OIL: Corn, cottonseed, peanut, and sesame; alternatives to olive. Sesame oil is particularly useful in sunscreens.

Herbs

(Any of the following herbs in tea-bag form, when moistened and placed on your eyelids, works wonders for tired eyes.)

CHAMOMILE: A healing agent extracted from the flowers of a European plant. Its tea is used as a rinse to enhance the luster of blond hair. A tonic and pain reliever. Has an applelike odor.

COMFREY: A healing plant root that promotes growth of healthy tissue and helps renew the skin. Its tea is used on skin.

GINSENG: The alleged wonder root of the Orient, where it is believed by many to be an aphrodisiac and cure for almost anything. Such claims have no basis in scientific fact. Also very expensive.

ROSEMARY: Used with sage as a hair conditioner and to control dandruff.

SAGE: Used with rosemary as a hair conditioner and to control dandruff. Has astringent and cleansing properties.

Cereals

BARLEY MEAL: Used in a mask as a soothing and healing agent.

BUCKWHEAT MEAL: Good for facial scrubs or in a mask in combination with antiseptics or astringents.

OATMEAL: Its coarse texture makes it very good for facial scrubs. Also makes a soothing mask. Whatever you do, DON'T BUY INSTANT!

Earths

FULLER'S EARTH: A claylike mineral that comes in many colors. Firms the skin when applied as a paste and allowed to dry.

KAOLIN: Also called white or china clay. A purer form of fuller's earth. Has an absorbent, shrinking, tightening effect on the skin when applied in a mask.

Spices

GINGER: The powdered root of a beautiful, exotic plant. An astringent, it stimulates blood flow when rubbed on the skin.

NUTMEG: The hard seed of a small tropical tree. Its oil is useful in hot footbaths.

Astringents and Antiseptics

ALCOHOL (RUBBING): A colorless, mildly aromatic fluid that creates a rosy glow when rubbed on the skin. EXTREMELY POISONOUS; DO NOT TAKE INTERNALLY.

ALUM: Used as an astringent for enlarged pores. Also used in styptic pencils for shaving nicks and in antiperspirants.

ALUMINUM ACETATE: Used in solutions as a very strong astringent. Also called Burow's solution.

HYDROGEN PEROXIDE: Used in dilute solution in water. Has a cleansing and germ-killing effect on skin. One of the gentlest antiseptics. (It is pleasant to watch it bubble.)

SODIUM PERBORATE: Dissolved in water, makes a good footbath.

SPIRITS OF CAMPHOR: Has a cooling effect on the skin. Contains soothing and healing compounds. Good for cold sores and to dry pimples. (Use only USP* grade, available in drugstores.)

IODINE SOLUTION: A strong antiseptic solution.

Cleansers and Soothing Agents

BICARBONATE OF SODA: Dissolved in water, makes a soothing wash for skin rashes. Has odor-absorbing properties.

BORAX: A super cleanser, skin softener, and body soak. Mixed with witch hazel, it makes a nice facial. (Use only USP grade, available in drugstores—not Forty Mule Team.)

MILK OF MAGNESIA: A skin-soothing agent.

VINEGAR: A weak 5 percent solution is an excellent astringent and a good cleanser. (Regular supermarket vinegar is a 5 percent solution.)

* USP is the abbreviation for "United States Pharmacopeia," which lists the legally recognized standards for drugs, is published, and periodically revised.

ZINC OXIDE: Has soothing, astringent, masking, and healing properties. Used in powder or ointment form.

Moisturizers

COCOA BUTTER: A fat derived from cocoa beans. Heals as it moistens. Use only in its pure form.

GLYCERIN: Having an affinity for water, acts as an antidrying agent. Keeps your skin from drying out. Great for chapped lips or hands.

Powders

CORNSILK POWDER: Used in masks and in face and bath powders.

CORNSTARCH: Used as a dusting powder or mixed in a bath to relieve dry, itchy skin.

TALC: Used in many cosmetics for its protective and slippery properties.

Waters

ALKANET SOLUTION: Made from the chips of a root soaked in witch hazel. Has astringent properties. A wonderful natural skin toner.

FRUIT WATERS: Used in masks, cleansers, toners, and other preparations.

ORANGE-FLOWER WATER: A solution of orange-flower oil in water. Used in perfume. Adds a lovely fresh smell and a quality of sparkle to skin.

ROSE WATER: A solution of oil distilled from rose flowers. Used mostly in colognes.

VEGETABLE WATERS: Used in masks, cleansers, and toners.

WITCH HAZEL: A water and alcohol solution of distilled extract of leaves and bark of the witch-hazel bush. An excellent freshener and astringent, hair rinse, a deodorant—you name it!

Lubricants

MINERAL OIL: A transparent, colorless, odorless, tasteless oil extracted from minerals. Rubbed on skin, it gives it a shiny protective, moisture-retaining film.

PETROLEUM JELLY: A good lubricant. Helps to soften and smooth the skin but may create a greasy feel.

TEXTURIZED LARD: A very sensual, smooth, odorless, colorless lubricant. An especially good skin softener.

RECIPES

Cleansers

Cleanser No. 1—Madame Christine Valmy's Washing Compound

½ cup kaolin
½ cup zinc oxide powder
½ cup pure soap flakes

- Mix dry ingredients thoroughly and keep in tightly closed jars.
- To use, mix 1 teaspoon with enough water to make a paste.
- Either leave on face 10 to 15 minutes or wash off right away.
- Don't scrub.
- Rinse with floods of water.
- Pat dry with fluffy towel.

Madame Valmy's Washing Compound, which is excellent for both men and women, will leave the skin with a matte finish, yet velvety and soft. Keep a jar of it in your office. It's great to use for a quick "fresh-up" to help you look your best for an important meeting or conference.

Cleanser No. 2—Comfrey Splendor

1½ ounces comfrey tea steeped overnight
1½ ounces rose water or orange-flower water
½ teaspoon borax crystals *Sodium Borate*

- Combine comfrey tea and whichever water you use.
- Add borax and shake to dissolve.
- Spray on skin as a fine mist, with a plant sprayer or atomizer.

This rinse is excellent for cleansing and relaxing the skin after a hard day at the office or out of doors.

Astringents

Astringent No. 1—A Hint of Autumn

1 pint broccoli water
Juice of ½ fresh lemon
4 drops spirits of camphor

• Shake all ingredients together in one of your beautiful bottles.
• Refrigerate until use.
• Pat liberally onto face with cotton square.
• Let dry naturally.
• Do not keep for more than 7 days.

Astringent No. 2—Midwinter's Warmth

1 ounce almond oil
2 ounces orange-flower water
½ teaspoon vinegar

• Mix together in a glass bottle.
• Warm bottle under hot running water.
• Shake to blend before using.
• Spray it on until skin is misty moist.
• Can be kept in refrigerator up to 3 weeks.

You can either let this astringent dry naturally on your skin or apply a moisturizer over the astringent while it is still moist.

Astringent No. 3—Hints of Spring

2 teaspoons witch hazel
¾ cup distilled water
1 teaspoon salt
⅛ teaspoon oil of wintergreen

• Dissolve salt in distilled water.
• Add witch hazel and oil of wintergreen.
• Put in bottle.
• Warm bottle under hot running water.
• Shake to blend before using.

• Pat it liberally on skin with cotton square, avoiding contact with mucous membranes.
• Let dry naturally.

This astringent is great for summer use when you've been out in the sun and need to feel cool. It's a wonderful body splash as well as a facial astringent.

Astringent No. 4—Summer Sport

2 tablespoons beer
1 tablespoon sugar

• Add sugar to beer.
• Swirl until beer foams and sugar dissolves.
• Apply to face with a cotton square. Also especially good for elbows, knees, and heels.
• Let dry naturally.

This is wonderful for summer use. In addition, the foam from warm, shaken beer makes an excellent cleanser.

Toners

Toner No. 1—Smooth Tone

1 ounce beet juice
3 ounces witch hazel

• Mix together in bottle.
• Keep cool in refrigerator until used.
• Apply to skin with cotton square.
• Let dry naturally.

This warm-weather toner is a good skin freshener.

Toner No. 2—Darkened Splendor

1 teaspoon alkanet root
4 ounces witch hazel

• Soak root in witch hazel until liquid takes on a deep red-brown color.
• Strain the liquid into a bottle.

• Discard the alkanet root.
• Apply to skin evenly with cotton squares.
• Let dry naturally.

This is an especially good toner for men. It is a natural coloring agent, good for darkening light skins slightly.

Toner No. 3—Juicy Roses

1 ounce fresh lemon juice
2 ounces rose water
¼ teaspoon iodine solution

• Combine ingredients in a bottle.
• Immerse bottle under hot running water to settle the ingredients.
• Shake well before use.
• Apply to skin sparingly with cotton square only where needed.
• Let dry naturally.
• Do not keep for more than 3 days.

This is a bleaching toner to be used for small red or darkened areas or around a scab where scar tissue forms.

Masks

Facial masks are wonderful pick-me-ups when you are feeling tired, low, or in need of some beauty. Leave masks on for from five to thirty minutes—until they dry thoroughly and crack on their own, or until they feel tight enough on your face.

Let your shower take the mask off, with medium-pressure warm water like heavy rain in summer. Don't scrub it off—let the water do the work. Rinse well. Remember that clay can look rinsed off when it isn't, so rinse especially well when you have clay in your mask.

All drawing masks can be used on your hands.

Mask No. 1—Basic

½ tablespoon fuller's earth
Yolk of 1 large egg
Liquid astringent

• Mix egg yolk and fuller's earth to a stiff paste.

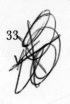

• Add astringent until paste is thin enough to spread easily.
• Smooth onto face.
• Relax while it works.

This is a great general "use-it-all-the-time" mask. For a little variety, use different color fuller's earth—it comes in white, buff, brown, green, olive, and blue.

Mask No. 2—Citrus Toner

Yolk of 1 large egg
Juice of ½ lemon or lime, or ¼ orange

• Beat egg yolk until it is fluffy.
• Blend in juice.
• Rub citrus peel on face as abrasive.
• Smooth onto face.
• Listen to light, airy music while it works.

This makes a transparent mask. (Another way to use citrus fruit as a toner is to freeze a lemon or lime in the ice compartment of your fridge. This breaks down the fiber of the peel, releasing into the white part under the skin a substance which you can rub on the face.)

Mask No. 3—Light California

1 overripe avocado
¼ cup buckwheat or barley meal

• Whip avocado pulp to a light puree.
• Add meal to make a smooth paste that will spread on easily.
• Smooth onto face.

This mask is especially good after any treatment that includes a medicated substance as blackhead or pimple repair.

Mask No. 4—Winter's Wonder

1 teaspoon sugar
½ teaspoon fresh lemon juice
1 tablespoon honey
1 teaspoon evaporated milk

• Dissolve sugar in lemon juice.

- Add milk.
- Stir in honey.
- Smooth onto face.
- Refrigerate any leftover.
- Do not keep for more than 3 days.

This mask is fabulous when your skin is exposed to very cold weather.

Mask No. 5—Complex Beauty

1 tablespoon flour
½ teaspoon fresh lemon juice
1 tablespoon lemon-scented cleansing lotion
½ teaspoon evaporated milk
Yolk of 1 large egg
1 tablespoon distilled water

- Make a paste with lemon juice and flour (or fuller's earth).
- Blend in cleansing lotion and milk until mixture is creamy.
- Beat egg yolk until fluffy and add to mixture.
- Place over low heat and cook, stirring constantly, until mixture thickens. (Do not overcook, or it will curdle.)
- Let cool before using.
- Smooth onto face.

This is the perfect mask for the hands as well as for the face. It takes time and effort but is well worth the trouble!

Mask No. 6—Honey-Lemon

1 tablespoon honey
White of 1 large egg
¼ teaspoon fresh lemon juice

- Blend egg white and honey.
- Add lemon juice.
- Smooth onto face.

This is a good greaseless, tightening mask, especially good for toning skin after shaving.

Mask No. 7—Garlic Gleam

1 packet active dry yeast
½ cup warm whole milk

1 teaspoon sugar

• Mix well and let stand one hour.

1 tablespoon yeast/milk/sugar mixture
2 5-grain perles of garlic oil

• Pierce garlic perles containing garlic oil with a needle and squeeze
    the oil into the yeast/milk/sugar mixture.
• Stir together well.
• Smooth onto face.

This mask is designed especially for dry skin. You may wish to be
alone when you use it, certainly not with a garlic-hater. Be brave—
I think garlic makes you sexy!

Mask No. 8—Browned Splendor

Yolk of 1 large egg
1 tablespoon fuller's earth
1 tablespoon lemon-scented cleansing lotion
¼ teaspoon vinegar

• Blend fuller's earth and egg yolk.
• Blend in cleansing lotion.
• Blend in vinegar to make smooth, fluffy paste.
• Smooth onto face.

This mask will have a deep-cleansing effect on your face. Use it
when you feel like cleansing away unpleasant thoughts.

Mask No. 9—Peeled Clean

2 teaspoons sugar
¼ cup fresh whole milk
½ teaspoon borax crystals

• Mix together.
• Smooth onto face.

This is a deep-cleansing mask, and you get to play the little peeling game to take it off.

Mask No. 10—California Heavy

2 tablespoons overripe avocado pulp
1 tablespoon evaporated milk

1 rounded tablespoon texturized lard or PABA (para-aminobenzoic acid) cream
6 drops fresh lemon juice
1 ground niacin tablet

• Warm avocado pulp over steam.
• Work milk and lard (or PABA cream) into the still steaming pulp.
• Add other ingredients for a fluffy, creamy mask.
• Smooth onto face immediately.

This is a rejuvenating mask—good for use in early spring to get rid of mature skin and make way for new cell growth.

Emollient

It's Bananas Eye Cream

1½ inches very ripe banana (brown, but not rotten)
1 teaspoon honey
¼ teaspoon fresh skimmed milk
Several drops fresh lemon juice

• Mash banana to smooth, even consistency.
• Blend in honey.
• Blend in milk and lemon juice.
• Use at once on eyelids and around eyes.
• What you do not use, throw away.

Use this cream when eyes are dark, puffy, or look and feel tired.

YOUR SPECIALS

Your specials include—
• Cell salts
• Special strategy recipes
• Wine soaks
• Put your best foot forward

Cell Salts

I use cells salts externally as soaks and recommend them as soaks for you—they could be a valuable addition to your apothecary. Use as directed on the packages. They are available at most health food stores.

These are the ones that I use:

CALCAREA FLUORICA (calcium fluoride) Found in bones and tooth enamel, and in the elastic fibers in skin, connective tissue, and vessel walls. Good for hard or thickened skins and for eczema.

CALCAREA PHOSPHORICA (calcium phosphate, phosphate of lime) Found in bones and teeth. Good for dry cold skin, wrinkles, and pimples.

CALCAREA SULPHURICA (calcium sulfate, gypsum, sulfate of lime) Found in skin, connective tissue, and blood. Good for boils, cuts, wounds, and bruises.

KALI MURIATICUM (potassium chloride) Essential for brain cell formation. Found in blood corpuscles, muscles, nerves, and intracellular fluid. Good for swollen boils and pimples containing pus.

KALI SULPHURICUM (potassium sulfate) Found principally in blood and also in epidermis. Good for pustular lesions. Also good for poison ivy.

KALI PHOSPHORICUM (potassium phosphate) Found principally in the brain and nerve cells. Good for wrinkled, withered-looking skin, itching skin, and eczema due to nervousness.

NATRUM SULPHURICUM (sodium sulfate) Found throughout the body in tissues and fluids. Good for swollen, stiff fingers; raw, sore palms; and tingling, painful skin.

NATRUM PHOSPHORICUM (sodium phosphate) Found in blood, muscles, nerves, brain cells, and intercellular fluids. Good for chafed skin, hives, and itchy ankles.

FERRUM PHOSPHORICUM (ferric phosphate) Found in every cell of the body; plentiful in red blood corpuscles. Good for fresh wounds, burning skin, and acne.

MAGNESIA PHOSPHORICA (magnesium phosphate) Found in nerves, muscles, and marrow of spine. Good for burning and stinging in corns and bunions, boils, and insect bites.

SILICEA (silicon dioxide) Traces found in hair, nails, and epidermis. Good for sensitive skin, itching, and acne.

Special Strategy Recipes

Pore Paste No. 1

1 teaspoon powdered alum
Yolk of 1 large egg
1 tablespoon barley meal
Juice of ½ fresh lemon
Whole milk

• Mix alum and barley meal and blend in egg yolk to make a paste.
• Add milk to thin the paste slightly.
• Add lemon juice and mix just before using.
• Smooth onto areas where pores are enlarged.

This paste is used for repair.

Pore Paste No. 2

1 teaspoon bicarbonate of soda
Camphor oil

• Moisten the bicarbonate of soda with enough oil to make a paste.
• Smooth onto areas where pores are enlarged.

This paste is to be used for maintenance after using Pore Paste No. 1.

Pore Paste No. 3

1 teaspoon powdered alum
1 ounce paraffin wax

• Melt paraffin.
• Stir in alum.
• Allow to cool.
• To use, remelt and apply before it is hot to areas where pores are enlarged.

Eye-Soak Wonder

1 ounce reduced potato water
1 ounce witch hazel

• To get reduced potato water, place 1 large clean baking potato in its skin in a small saucepan with enough water to cover it about halfway. Add ½ teaspoon fresh lemon juice. Cook it covered, gently boiling, until it is soft. Continue adding water to keep the potato half covered. When potato is done, remove and continue boiling the water until it is reduced to half its volume.
• Mix the potato water and witch hazel.
• Moisten eyelids and entire area around eyes with a cotton square soaked with the solution.
• Place one cotton square moistened with the solution under each eye and let it stay for 10 minutes.

Stretch-Mark Astringent

2 ounces fresh lemon juice
1 ounce rose water
½ ounce vinegar

• Mix ingredients well.
• Store in glass spray bottle in refrigerator.
• Spray on stretch marks.
• Let dry naturally.
• Then massage area with your favorite oil.

Use the astringent daily until stretch marks fade. Don't be discouraged—it may take as long as 6 months.

Drink for Ashy Skin

1 tablespoon soybean pellets with lecithin
1 teaspoon garlic oil (equivalent to 14 large perles)
Honey to taste

• Mix ingredients.
• Drink neat or stirred into a hot beverage or warm milk.
• Take at night before going to bed.

This rejuvenating drink will bring back a glow to the skin. It will also liven up your liver.

Bleaching Mask

1 heaping tablespoon warm boiled white potato
½ tablespoon lard
1 teaspoon sugar/milk mixture (see below)

* To make sugar/milk mixture, add ¼ teaspoon sugar to 3 teaspoons whole milk.
* Cream lard and potato together thoroughly.
* Add sugar/milk mixture.
* Blend it well, fluffing up as much as possible.
* Apply only for spot bleaching.

Wine Soaks

For a luxurious splurge, take a wine soak! Here's what to do:

* Pour all of a 3-liter bottle of red wine in a tub of hot water.
* Add 4 ounces Epsom salts.
* Soak for 20 minutes while sipping any mulled wine.
* Rinse off in shower.

Put Your Best Foot Forward

Poor feet . . . what you do put them through . . . shoes too tight, heels too high, soles with no padding! Walking all day on concrete, discoing to the wee hours!

Have pity on them. After all, if they stop, so do you! And in your life, too, these two little guys, which have one quarter of all the bones in your body, will probably walk over 70,000 miles!!

Tips on Foot Care

* Always soak your feet in water at body temperature or colder.
* When your feet are tired or aching, soak them in warm water with foot soap, then pumice the pressure points with a circular motion.
* If your feet itch from dryness, apply calamine lotion.
* Have as many white socks as you have face cloths. Put foot cream on your city-tired feet at night, then put on your white socks, to massage and to condition your feet.

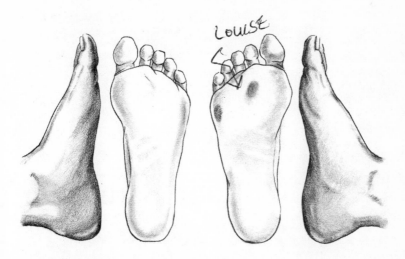

Using a circular motion, rub the pressure areas (ball of foot and heel) of your feet with pumice.

• Remove surface dryness with moisturizer. Massage well into feet. Leave on to cool. Rinse. Follow with a cold cocoa-butter massage to leave your feet dancing pretty.

If you have corns or calluses, see a podiatrist. Never try to remove them yourself. To maintain callus-free feet, use pumice with soap daily. Pumicing is also useful on rough heels and for removing embedded dirt.

3

Your Bathroom

MAKING A PLACE FOR PERSONAL CARE

BELIEFS in the absolving powers of bathing stem from the earliest cultures of dark-complexioned peoples and survive today in Hindu India and in Bali where the outdoor baths are a part of temple architecture and religious practice.

Excavations at Knossos, the ruined four-thousand-year-old center of Cretan civilization, revealed what is believed to be the site of the earliest bathroom. Bathing facilities were an important part of the ancient Greek and Roman civilizations. President Millard Fillmore, in 1850, had the distinction of putting the first bathtub in the White House and was criticized for wasting public funds.

Associated with the bathroom throughout its history have been the notions of privacy and quiet as well as of cleansing and grooming. You, too, must bear in mind in decorating your bathroom that it is not only a place where you frequently exercise your beauty treatment ritual but also a place where private introspection . . . meditation . . . and total relaxation should be possible.

For today's sophisticate, the bathroom should once again become a retreat from the wear and tear of one's frantic yet fascinating lifestyles—a place of free communing with the spirits. In this setting, one can concentrate on evolving into that beautiful image one wishes to project.

Unfortunately, the standard American bathroom of today is criminally small and inadequate. It has become the "powder room," the room of the "quick wash," the toilet, instead of the total pampering room. How strange this seems when our living rooms, parlors, dining rooms, playrooms, and bedrooms are not only spacious but also embellished with fine furniture, rich carpeting, and decorative paintings and ornaments. We have turned our attention from body care and pampering to superficial pleasures and trappings.

For the true seeker of beauty, it is time to recapture the bathroom as a Pierian's private sanctuary for pampering—as a mini-salon—from the commonplace bathroom which has a totally functional design.

Here's how to do just that!

The Equipment

Your bathroom's equipment probably consists of the basic four:

• Bathtub/shower
• Toilet
• Basin
• Medicine cabinet

Which means you probably don't have enough shelf space, the right kind of shower head, or a nice place to soak your feet.

So . . . a few investments:

If your medicine cabinet is like eight of every ten, it has two sliding doors. Remove one door so you can place often-used cosmetics within easy reach.

Put up some shelving where you can. Glass is best since it gives a clean, sparkling appearance (and since your glass bottles and jars will look even more invitingly beautiful on glass shelves!).

Buy and attach to shower outlet a telephone-type shower head with hose—one that can be adjusted for different types of water flow.

If your bathtub has sliding doors, remove them and hang a

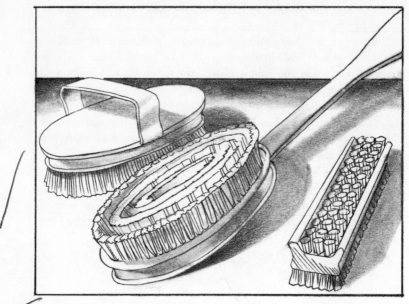

Brushes. Left to right: Body brush, body brush with handle for the shower, nail-and-foot brush.

shower curtain instead. You can't attach anything to sliding doors; you can't reach other things you want when you're in the shower; and their tracks accumulate grime.

Keep a metal pan handy, large enough to hold your feet comfortably without touching your toes or heels, to use for soaking your feet.

The Decor

Your bathroom should be painted in pastel or neutral colors—no deep colors or tones, please! Any highlighting or contrasting paint should be in a glossy white. The color you choose should be partly but not totally flattering to you.

Lighting

A lot of lighting of varying types is ideal for establishing your optimum beauty environment:

Begin with the overhead lighting. Install a screw-type fixture for a 125-watt bulb with a "dimmer" switch.

Surround the mirror by lights so you can see any problem areas on your face.

Install a heat-light fixture, to be used when additional heat penetration or a drying light is needed.

Mirrors

Ah . . . the more the better! Have a floor-length mirror, a wide true-image mirror, a hand-held mirror that reflects regular image on one side and a magnified image on the other, and a round mirror surrounded by lights.

Floor Covering

Rubber matting—the type with soft, close-packed little spikes—is the best floor covering for the bathroom. In addition to trapping spilled water, it is very soothing for tired feet—gives them a stimulating massage while you simply stand there and move around completing your beauty treatment!

Shelves and Storage

As I've already said, put up some extra glass shelves to hold your cosmetic apothecary.

Have your storage space and shelves convenient to your reach and place your items so that the ones you use most are nearest to where you will use them.

Crowning Touch

Music. Choose soothing instrumental music for your stereo, to suit what you're doing.

Don't allow any talking during your ritual beauty time . . . and that includes a radio announcer, a singer, or your mate!

Scent. Choose mood-type scents like incense and natural aromatic burning oils, to perfume the air so as to create tranquility and relaxation.

Don't have floral sprays raining down on you. If you want a floral reminder, put one or two of your favorite flowers in a vase or choose the flower of your birth month or that of the month it now is:

Month	Birth Flower
January	Carnation
February	Violet
March	Jonquil
April	Sweet pea
May	Lily of the valley
June	Rose
July	Larkspur
August	Gladiolus
September	Aster
October	Calendula
November	Chrysanthemum
December	Narcissus

Plants. If you're a plant lover, you'll want to share your beauty room with your living green friends. Keep to the small-size varieties and only ones that like lots of water and high humidity.

If You're the Lucky One Who Can Build Your Own

If you're building your own house, you can have the pampering room of your dreams. And by all means do . . . splurge a lot!

Tell your architect you want a large room with special features. Take a hint from the Japanese and have a tile floor with a drain so it won't matter in the least if you get gallons of water at a time on the floor.

Have the toilet closed off in a tiny room of its own so it won't detract from your pampering.

Have a sunken oval tub large enough for you and someone else. And have whirlpool spouts in that tub.

Have a basin large enough (and high enough) for you to immerse your face without having to fear a brain concussion from the faucets.

Have a shower stall with three or four shower heads at different heights and on opposite walls, as well as a hose-and-telephone-type shower head.

Have a bidet installed for quick, easy, and hygienic body cleansing.

Have full-length mirrors facing each other.

Have floor-to-ceiling windows on the north side, if possible. Artists agree that a north light is the best one to paint by—having no glare, it shows the colors of paints and the lineaments of the object being painted most faithfully.

4

Treatments Just for You

THE PERFECT TIME for initiating beauty rejuvenation is spring —for those who are joined to all living things there is hope. Each season of the year places unique demands on your skin because of temperature, wind, cold, sun, and humidity changes. During spring and summer your body responds to heat and sun by relaxing your pores to provide cooling by perspiration. Perspiration also acts as a kind of natural cleaner of the skin. However, any new season is the perfect time for you to embark upon your Seven-Day Beauty Plan since your purpose, of course, is to create seasons for your own complexion, head to toe.

YOUR SEVEN-DAY BEAUTY PLAN

Day 1	A One-day Fast and a Professional Pampering
Day 2	Design Your Treatment
Day 3	Stock Your Apothecary
Day 4	Prepare Your Cosmetics
Day 5	Begin Your Regimen
Day 6	Massage and Bath-treatment Time
Day 7	Have Your Hair Styled, Buy a New Outfit, Go out on the Town

But before you start your plan there are a few things you should consider.

What Type Skin Do I Have?

Although all skin has the same fundamental reaction, dark skins are perhaps better adapted to extreme summer sun and heat than light skins because dark skins are richer in pigmentation and sebaceous-gland activity.

Skin shades of black people vary considerably. They may be—

> jet black
> black/gray
> light or dark chestnut ✓
> gray/red
> brown/red
> bronze
> **red**
> blue-black/purple

There are three basic skin types, and each requires a somewhat different beauty care plan:

> *oily skin*
> *dry skin*
> *normal skin*

✓

The Skin Type Test: Do this test in the summer when your skin oils flow freely.

First, look at your skin. Excessively oily skin shines—you can see the oil. Excesively dry skin looks dull. It feels tight and has a tendency to become chapped and to peel.

Next, place a silk cloth, a piece of onionskin, or a piece of coarse vellum paper over your entire face and gently press it onto your skin. This will show you where your oily areas are. If the entire cloth is oily, chances are good that that is your skin type.

Dry skin is indicative of an overly acid-producing skin, oily skin an overly alkaline-producing skin. The purpose of skin care is to neutralize both oily and dry conditions so that all skin may be treated as normal.

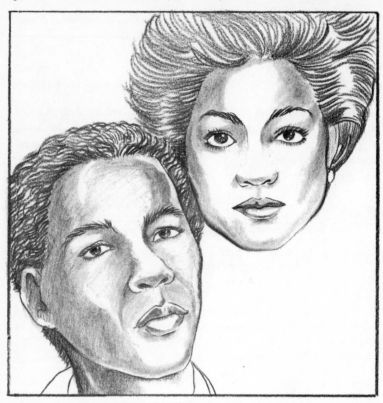

Ashy-appearing skin is often a result of one of the following four things: (1) extreme shower or tub-bath water temperature—either too hot or too cold—when the water first comes in contact with your body; (2) mild skin shocks from going from water temperature to room temperature; (3) failure to rinse off cleansing agents well enough; (4) drying your skin with towels too briskly.

Itching skin often means sensitive skin—that you have used the wrong cleansing agent, one that dries into the pores; or that wet skin has not been properly dried.

A good way to improve your overall body tones is to lie flat on your back on the floor and do keep breathing exercises for three minutes.

Care Demands by Skin Type

Although the basic steps are the same for all skin types, they are not always repeated in sequence since the demands of oily skin care differ from those of dry skin care.

For oily skin, the key is deep cleansing and it should be gentle but frequent. Alternate soft complexion brushes with cloths.

For dry skin, the key is protective moisturizing and it should be adequate as well as frequent.

Seasonal and Geographical Variations

Oily Skin. Brushing refines skin surface textures.

Spring: Steaming and deep pore cleansing every day in every region.

Summer: Steaming and deep pore cleansing every day in every region.

Autumn: Steaming and deep pore cleansing twice a week in the North and East, three times a week in the South and West.

Winter: Steaming and deep pore cleansing three times a week in every region.

Dry Skin. A thin application of any natural oil is a basic need.

Spring: Steaming and deep pore cleansing three times a week in the North and East, twice a week in the South and West.

Summer: Steaming and deep pore cleansing four times a week in the North and East, three times a week in the South and West; when tanning, every day after sun exposure in every region.

Autumn: Steaming and deep pore cleansing twice a week in every region.

Winter: Deep pore cleansing once a week followed by steaming in every region. For days when the temperature is below freezing, an extra thin application of any natural oil to form a glaze is a must before going out.

Normal Skin. All regions require the same.

Spring: Steaming and deep pore cleansing twice a week.

Summer: Steaming and deep pore cleansing three times a week.

Autumn: Steaming and deep pore cleansing twice a week.

Winter: Steaming and deep pore cleansing once a week.

Now you know your skin type and what special care demands it has. You are ready to start your Seven-Day Beauty Plan.

DAY 1—A ONE-DAY FAST AND A PROFESSIONAL PAMPERING

Start your beauty plan on your day according to numerology. Your number is the date of your birth, reduced to a single digit. For example, if you were born on the twenty-fifth of any month, your number is seven. You get the number by adding together the two digits—$2 + 5 = 7$. If the sum is greater than a single digit when you add the digits—say, you were born on the twenty-ninth: $2 + 9 = 11$—you add the digits in the sum—$1 + 1 = 2$—and two is your number.

On your first day, go on a one-day purifying fast, eating and drinking nothing but eight to ten large glasses of water. You can add a slice of lemon or lime to allay your fasting thoughts as you look ahead to a day of water only.

Visit external care doctors—for example, a chiropractor or a podiatrist for their corrective pampering suggestions.

Visit a facial salon and have a professional treatment so you can start off with a clean skin surface. The skin care specialist can help answer any questions you have about your treatment regimen and the products you should use.

DAY 2—DESIGN YOUR TREATMENT

The Basic Steps

Regardless of season and weather conditions, there are four basic steps your skin care needs in its year-round consistent program of care.

> Pore opening
> Cleansing/lubricating
> Pore closing and toning
> Protection/balance

The *first step* is to open your pores. One of the most effective ways is a facial steaming, which relaxes pores, pushes out impurities, and softens skin by providing necessary moisture.

The best way to steam your face at home is to put herbs in a heat-proof glass bowl, pour boiling distilled water over them, drape a towel over your head, and hold your face over the steam. Use 2 tablespoons of herbs to 1 quart of water. For any skin, the best steams are—

> relaxing and invigorating—peppermint
> relaxing and stimulating—thyme or lavender
> relaxing and cleansing—rosemary

A second way is to use hot-towel compresses. The best compresses are made with terry cloth towels.

Another way is to steam your face over gently simmering vegetables, also under a draped towel. If you use this method, be careful not to hold your face too near the flame.

The *second step* is to give your face a thorough deep cleansing. This can be accomplished with soaps, lotions, and creams designed to deep-cleanse or with masks, facial scrubs, or facial rinses; see the recipes in Chapter 2. The Comfrey Splendor (p. 29) is an excellent cleanser; comfrey can also be added to any mask recipe. Comfrey is recognized as a promoter of new skin growth by means of its component allantoin. Comfrey masks will moisturize while they are cleansing.

The *third step* is to close your pores. This you do with any of the astringents you have made from the recipes in Chapter 2. Remember that your choice of astringents depends on the season.

The *fourth step* is to protect your skin until the next treatment. This is accomplished through the use of round-the-clock moisturizing agents—emollients to give your skin its protective layer.

These four steps vary in their frequency depending on your skin type and on seasonal differences. As you develop your beauty plan, your ideal routine will evolve.

DAY 3—STOCK YOUR APOTHECARY

Try to make this a day when you are not busy doing anything else or when you are not working so you can spend the entire day beauty shopping. The basic American beauty always has a supply of cold cream and petroleum jelly; the very chic has carbolated petroleum jelly.

DAY 4—PREPARE YOUR COSMETICS

Place all your cosmetic ingredients on the shelves where they are convenient for your use.

Prepare whatever cosmetics you will need. Refrigerate them if necessary or store them in beautiful bottles on your bathroom shelves.

DAY 5—BEGIN YOUR REGIMEN

Cleansing. Begin your cleansing regimen in the evening. Then alternate cleansings, some in the morning, some in the evening.

First, splash lots and lots of water on your face or pat it on with one of your washcloths. Use a cloth only once, then wash it. Begin with cool water, then lukewarm water. This moisturizes and softens your skin.

Cleanse your face.

Rinse cleanser off thoroughly with lots of water.

Next pat your face dry with a freshener- or astringent-soaked cotton square.

At bedtime:

Apply night cream to damp face. (Creams find better levels of penetration on predampened skin.)

Apply special-strategy ointments to areas that need it—for enlarged pores, pimples, and cleaned blackhead areas.

In the morning:

When you wake up, spray lots and lots of mineral water on your face—first cool, then lukewarm.

Apply freshener or astringent to your face with a presoaked cotton square.

Apply day cream when skin is still damp from freshener or astringent.

Apply makeup if you wish.

Follow this routine morning and evening.

DAY 6—MASSAGE AND BATH-TREATMENT TIME

Today go and have a professional body massage.

Then take a luxurious soak—either in a bath salts soak, an herbal bath, or a fresh-flower soak.

If you opt for the herbal bath, choose the herb to suit your mood and whichever you feel you need. *Chamomile* moisturizes, heals, and stimulates circulation. *Pine* is calming. *Comfrey* has astringent qualities. *Eucalyptus* is antiseptic and cools.

To get the most from the herbs, tie a handful in a linen cloth or in a washcloth and boil it in a saucepan of water for a few minutes.

Then pour the water (and the bag) into your bath water.

If you want to relax, have your bath water warm to body temperature; if you want stimulation, try the water colder.

If you plan to cast magic upon yourself when you soak, set afloat fresh flowers in the language of the Goddess of Beauty: *Variegated tulip* for beautiful eyes. *China rose* for beauty always new. *Lady's slipper* for beauty capricious. *Flower-of-an-hour* (*hibiscus*) for beauty delicate. *American cowslip* for beauty divine. *Glory-flower* for beauty glorious. *Stock* for beauty lasting. *Calla lily* for beauty magnificent. *Clematis* for mental beauty. *Throatwort* for beauty neglected. *Laburnum* for beauty pensive. *French honeysuckle* for beauty rustic. *Burgundy rose* for beauty unconscious. *American red rose* if beauty is your only attraction.

DAY 7—HAVE YOUR HAIR STYLED, BUY A NEW OUTFIT, GO OUT ON THE TOWN

This is the perfect time for the new beautiful you to have a new hair style. Tell your hairdresser it's a new you being worked on.

New hair style . . . new beauty care . . . lovely skin . . . lovely spirit . . . deserve a lovely new clothing look, too. Remember, the color you choose will put a glow on your aura.

Go show everyone BEAUTIFUL NEW YOU!!

SPECIAL CARE

Children

Children's skin care should not be neglected but should be simple.

From birth to puberty—mineral water and oil cleansing from head to toe and additional oiling to areas where hair will grow, to soften the skin and help keep it supple, are in order.

In cold climates, apply lots of oil to children's skin. In warm climates, brush on powder to protect their skin's moisture balance.

Remember that skin care habits—poor ones as well as good ones —will be established in childhood.

Adolescents

Pimples often plague teenagers, particularly boys, and can be a source of embarrassment and concern for them. In addition to regular cleansing an adolescent may find the following special strategies useful:

Use pure castile soap, pine tar soap, or a pure unscented soap for deep pore cleansing.

Clean pimples themselves by applying slight pressure all around with a cotton-wrapped fingertip soaked with therapeutic solution.

Aging Skin

Maintaining one's weight after age thirty helps prevent skin from aging prematurely.

Aging skin requires more moisture. It requires heavier creams, more moisturizing, and more softening.

Aging skin also requires toning lotions to smooth and even change skin tones.

If skin is sallow or drab, toners help bring color back to the skin. Several drops of a good toner added to any mask is very helpful.

If your wrinkles bother you, consider plastic surgery for your eyes or a face lift, as described in detail in Chapter 5.

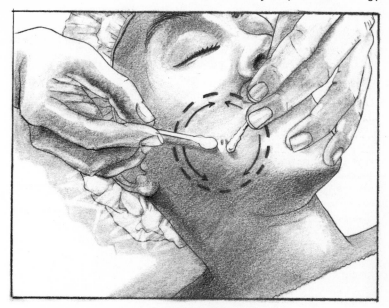

First step for removing blackheads or pimples.

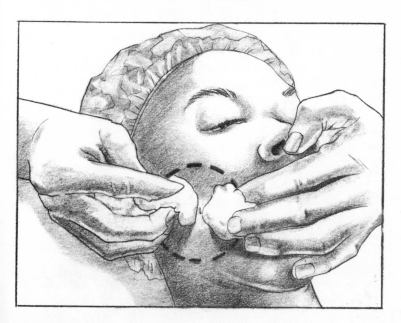

Second step. After the head is removed, surrounding area is massaged with cotton balls.

Bleaching as an Art

Most dark-complexioned persons have, at one time or another, areas or spots which become darker than their surrounding areas. Dark spots may result from touching pimples with dirty fingernails or fingertips or from trying to remove blackheads on a not-yet-cleansed face. Dark spots may appear when a wound heals, around the holes of pierced ears, from aging, and so on. To most of us, these spots are unsightly and we want to be rid of them as fast as possible.

That's usually quite easily done!

For only small, slightly darker spots, an application of fresh lemon juice has a bleaching effect if applied daily.

For very large darker areas, the best bleaching treatment is to sun-darken your entire body first so nature takes over and peels off some pigment. This is called "retoning."

HAND TREATMENT

Your hands say so much about you. There they are—gesturing, caressing, expressing, caring. Everyone sees them. And they portray the artistic you. So give them loving care.

Use a Honey-Lemon Mask (recipe on p. 34) on your hands. Leave it on long enough for it to harden. Then rinse it off with cool gently running water.

Spread Mask No. 5, Complex Beauty (p. 34), on your hands to give them a rebirth. After the mask has been on for twenty minutes, rinse it off with cool running water.

DRAB SKIN NO MORE

Use these procedures on your face twice a week if your skin seems drab for as long as you feel you need them.

Scrub Away the Drab

Cleanse with whichever of these formulas is correct for you:

Oily skin. Mix table salt with enough buttermilk to make a grainy mixture.

Dry skin. Blend the contents of one vitamin A capsule into a half cup of sour cream.

Normal skin. Same as above with plain yogurt instead of sour cream.

Steam open your pores over a bowl of hot herbal tea.

Spray your face with a mixture of ½ skimmed milk and ½ chamomile tea which has been cooled in the refrigerator.

Massage your face gently with heavy cream.

Scrub away dead surface cells. First, squeeze the juice from ½ a lemon; remove the pulp. Mix 2 tablespoons plain yogurt with the lemon pulp and enough oatmeal to make the mixture gritty. Pack the mixture into the lemon rind until it is full; wrap it in wet cheesecloth and secure with a rubber band. Work this over your face for 5 minutes. Remove traces of the scrub with damp washcloth.

Spray again with the milk/tea mixture.

Once a week, apply a mixture of ½ cup yogurt and 1½ teaspoons lemon juice to your face and leave on overnight.

Mask Away the Drab

Cleanse skin with a mild, nonoily cleanser.

Embryonic Peel-off. Crack open 3 eggs, remove the contents, and store. You only need the shells. Carefully peel off the membrane that clings to the inside of the shell, in as large pieces as possible. Smooth membrane pieces onto your face, concentrating on lined areas, large pores on cheeks, chin, and nose. Leave membrane pieces in place till they dry.

If your skin is oily, remove the membrane pieces by gently polishing your face with a pumice.

If your skin is dry, coat your face with a layer of a vegetable oil, and then use a pumice sponge.

Pasting. If your skin is oily, apply a paste of cornmeal and water on your face. Massage with a complexion brush and remove the cornmeal. If your skin is dry, apply a vegetable oil on your face. Massage with a complexion brush and leave on a half hour.

Paraffin Mask. Melt 1 ounce of paraffin wax in top of double boiler till it is of liquid consistency. Apply to face with paint brush. It should still be warm, but TEST WITH YOUR FINGER UNTIL YOU'RE SURE IT ISN'T SO HOT IT WILL BURN YOUR SKIN. Apply wax generously—warm paraffin forms a thin seal that pinpoints lines, wrinkles and blemishes.

Heat a metal spatula by running it back and forth across a pot of hot water until it is just warm, not too hot. Press gently over whole face, concentrating on trouble spots.

Pull off wax in big pieces as soon as it solidifies after spatula treatment.

Rinse your face with cold water, then pat on freshener or astringent.

GOOD-BYE STRETCH MARKS

If there was magic in cosmetic skin care it would rid your body of the stretch marks caused by weight gains, having babies, tight stressed skin, body building, and so on.

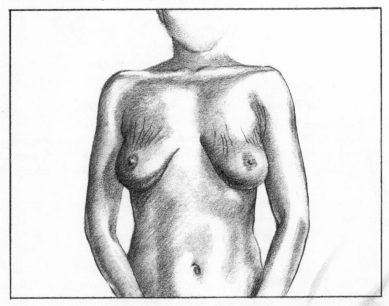

Massage early stretch marks with a downward motion after area has been warmed by a shower bath and/or massaged with oil.

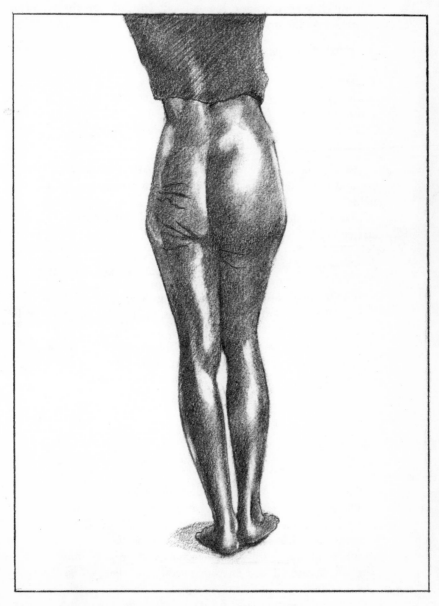

Use circular motion massage on these stretch-mark areas.

Constant skin conditioning is a way to cope with stretch marks. Too much soap cleansing is not good. Instead, use the following treatment on the stretch mark area:

Thorough cleansing with superfatted cleanser or textured cleansing cloth.

Loofah massage to increase circulation.

Daily spraying with Stretch-Mark Astringent (see p. 39) for stimulation and tone.

Daily body-oil massage applied while the astringent is still damp and tingling, to soften the elastic fibers.

It takes about six months for stretch marks to fade away in winter and about three months during the summer, when the sun can help.

Above all, don't despair . . . time heals all wounds . . . even stretch marks.

THE SOFT WAY TO TAN YOUR SKIN

We all know the healing and toning benefits of salt water and the sun. For the best tan and the safest, moderation of course is the key.

And for those most in the know, the very best tan comes from lying on a louvered platform over an outdoor hot tub to allow the steam to flow over you as the sun performs its wonder.

How to Do It

Over your outdoor hot tub or by the sea, remember that softening the skin before and after exposure to the sun makes the tan last longer.

First take a brisk shower in body-temperature water.

Then pat yourself dry with your tanning lotion to which you have added a few drops of Toner No. 3, Juicy Roses (see p. 32).

Spray on a table salt solution mixed with water.

While still damp, oil yourself heavily with tropical tanning lotion and rub texturized lard on your knees, your elbows, and the backs of your hands.

Lie down in the sun on your platform over a hot tub on each side of your body for 7 minutes several times a week between 7:30 A.M. and 11 A.M. when the outdoor temperature is about 75° F. and the humidity over 50 percent.

Follow each tanning session by a tub soak with added water softeners.

WATER WORKS

The water you use on your complexion should be soft—that is to say, free from minerals. To tell whether or not it is soft, do this: Run a basin full of water; make a lather with a pure unscented soap. If it lathers easily, the water is soft; if it does not lather easily, the water is hard.

If your water is hard, consider purchasing a water-softening device you can put onto the faucet. Or use water-softening bath salts; most chain drugstores carry such salts, at a reasonable price. You can also soften water by adding Epsom salts.

On a scale of 1 to 10 for soft-to-hard water, the major cities rank as follows:

New York	1
Washington	2
Baltimore	2
Detroit	3
Chicago	3
Boston	3
Philadelphia	4
Atlanta	5
Newark	5
San Francisco	5
Houston	5
Dallas	6
Los Angeles	9

Collect country rain or forest rain water in a 4-ounce bottle and seal it with a cork. Keep it chilled and use it as an eye rinse for those very special evenings when bright eyes are a must.

AND NOW FOR SOME FINAL BEAUTY HINTS

1. Have a salon facial once a month for rejuvenation.

2. A natural fabric moistened with fresh beet juice makes a rosy rouge for your face.

3. Eat a lot of apples when they are in season.

4. Keep silk or cotton gloves under your pillow. At night, put body oil on your hands, put on the gloves, and wear all night to soften your hands while you sleep.

5. Drink lots of water.

6. Wear natural fibers. They let your skin breath.

7. Be elegant at all times. It is basic for any glamorous person.

8. Create seasonal complexions by changing your cosmetic skin care with each season.

9. Use only one corrective cosmetic at a time to get rid of a skin problem.

10. Have a professional oil body massage once a month.

11. Pluck your eyebrows, holding tweezers at an angle. This will keep short stubs from showing up so quickly.

12. Soak a slice of lemon in water for your beauty drink.

13. Listen to Mozart when you use a facial mask.

14. Get a beauty secret of your own and don't tell anyone. Every great beauty has one.

5

When You
Need Outside Help

ALTHOUGH most of us are reasonably pleased with our looks, it is not narcissistic to want to improve our appearance. The growing pride and strength we take in being black are strong motivations to improve our looks, our image. There are few among us, male or female, who do not emit an inner glow when we feel we are looking well. An unsightly scar, a particularly flat nose, or protruding ears may mar this image needlessly. Many such flaws may be improved through reconstructive or cosmetic surgery. In this chapter I will show you how to let the art of surgery remake a feature into one which your genetic heritage didn't give you. The material is presented for information only and is not a recommendation.

RECONSTRUCTIVE VS. COSMETIC SURGERY

Although the two are parallel and inseparable in the particular patient, reconstructive surgery is considered to be surgery to repair disfigurements resulting from accident or injury. Cosmetic surgery refers to elective correction of a displeasing nose, lips, or other feature.

RECONSTRUCTIVE SURGERY

The Battle-scar Days Are Over

Scar production is the body's method of repairing itself. Any breach of the skin (or of other parts of the body, for that matter) results in scar-tissue formation.

How Scars Form. A scar is composed of collagen, a complex protein molecule that is produced rapidly by specialized cells at the injury site as the body's building block of repair. In a simple cut that is properly treated and heals without complications, the collagen is present from about the third day after the injury, builds up to a maximum in about forty days, then matures and strengthens to "heal" the wound.

What you see develop is a fine red line, which, after six to ten weeks, gradually fades to become a lighter line than its surrounding skin because it has no pigment.

In some people, scar formation is less orderly. Collagen is overproduced, leaving a thick, red, raised scar, of one of two types —hypertrophic or keloid.

Hypertrophic scars are usually wide, red scars which are raised above the surrounding skin surface. They are frequently associated with areas of tension—across joints such as elbows or knees or after injuries in which there has been great tissue loss or inadequate treatment.

Keloid scars are characterized by an excessive overgrowth of dense scar tissue, so much so that it is disfiguring. Even the most innocuous skin injury—a pierced ear or a small scratch—can result in an irregular, cauliflowerlike growth. In addition to being unsightly, keloid scars in certain areas such as the mouth or eyelid may actually interfere with function.

Although the cause of keloid scars is not known, they seem to be due to continued unchecked collagen production.

Dark-skinned Caucasians, Orientals, and blacks have a higher incidence of keloid scar formation. Although keloid scars are more difficult to manage surgically, in most cases they can be improved. To avoid these types of scar formations or to lessen their long-lasting effects, a person who has any injury more than $\frac{1}{16}$ of an inch in depth should get medical treatment. Neglect and poor treatment often result in bleeding, infection, and overwhelming tissue damage that can interfere with the surgeon's ability to minimize the final scar.

Some Considerations About Scars You Should Know

Alas . . . that scar is permanent. The first and foremost general consideration about scar surgery is that no operative procedure will eliminate or remove the scar entirely. Even with the most careful plans and skilled technique, when the surgeon joins together the two edges of fresh skin he or she must seal the union with collagen . . . or scar tissue. It is possible there will be an improvement and the magnitude of the injury minimized.

Don't expect skin grafts. The second consideration is that skin grafts are used rarely in scar correction. Many ask why the troubled area simply cannot be resurfaced with normal skin . . . back to the same basic principle—the healer and scar-maker collagen. When the graft is joined with normal tissue, the body forms a scar. Of course, in a major injury, such as a deep burn, when tissue destruction has been excessive, a skin graft may be the only answer. But for the small yet troublesome scar of the cheek or forehead, grafting has no place. Scar revision is the answer instead.

What scar . . . what revision . . . or, the good-looking scar. When a plastic surgeon looks at a scar, the following considerations are germane:

A scar which is elevated, or raised above the surrounding skin, can be reduced.

A scar which is depressed, or lower than the surrounding tissue, can be raised.

A wide scar can be narrowed.

An irregular or zigzag scar sometimes can be straightened.

A conspicuous scar—sometimes its direction can be changed to a direction or place where it is less conspicuous. For example, a vertical scar of the forehead may be changed to run parallel to the horizontal folds or a scar of the inner cheek may be moved into the crease running from the mouth to the nose.

These simple considerations cover the bulk of scar revision surgery and can make the scar on your face look much better.

Once the Decision Is Made About Surgery, Whom Do You Go to and What Happens?

So you've decided to do something to improve that ugly (at least, you see it that way) scar. How do you go about it?

I advise you to first consult a makeup artist who is expert at providing you the look you will have.

Take photos of the "old you" and the "new you" and compare what you see.

Wear your new look as often as you can to see how you like it; how it makes you feel about yourself; and how others react.

Now you're ready to choose and consult a plastic surgeon who'll help you become the face you wish to be. How do you find the right one?

Try to find someone who has had a satisfying surgical experience or ask someone whose new look you like who their surgeon is.

Ask your family physician for a referral.

Call the county medical society for a list of referrals.

Contact American Society of Plastic and Reconstructive Surgeons:

Suite 800
29 East Madison Street
Chicago, Illinois 60602
(312) 641-0593

Next . . . Your Consultation

So now you've chosen a plastic surgeon, scheduled the consultation appointment, and gone for the consultation.

Explain to the surgeon what bothers you about the scar.

The surgeon will: take a brief medical history; examine the scar you want revised and perhaps other scars you have; give you an estimate of likely improvement to help you make your decision.

Having considered the surgeon's findings, you may then decide whether or not to go ahead with the scar revision. If the surgeon estimates a 10 percent improvement as likely, the cost and inconvenience may be unjustifiable. If the surgeon estimates a 50 percent or greater improvement as likely, you may think surgery is justified and you make an appointment for the operation.

The Surgery Itself

Preoperative preparations. Follow whatever preparations the surgeon advises before the day of surgery. These may include vitamin therapy, special soaps and cleansing, and/or facials.

The day or surgery arrives and you go to the office surgical suite or hospital. Depending on your surgeon's and your own preference, you will have either a local or general anesthetic. Whichever you have, you will feel no pain during the surgery.

You will have sutures (stitches) and you may or may not have dressings or bandages. Be sure to follow the surgeon's instructions about whether or not to keep the surgery site covered.

Now for the Hard Part . . . A Lot of Patience

During the first twenty-four to forty-eight hours you may feel pain. The pain normally will be relieved by mild to moderate pain medicines. If it is not, contact your surgeon. While you're in pain, try to think beautiful thoughts about the new you.

The sutures and dressings will be removed early (to prevent suture marks) and the wound may be taped for several weeks to minimize tension on the suture line.

If your scar is hypertrophic, the treatment will involve steps to limit scar production, such as surgical techniques with minimal tension; careful postsurgical monitoring; and sometimes injection with a steroid-type drug to reduce the tendency for the scar to recur.

If your scar is keloid, the treatment will be more complex. The revision is more conservative. (Usually, it is not practical to alter keloid scar direction or position since additional scarring is likely. Most of the suturing is below the skin and any skin sutures are removed early since the skin suture itself may leave another keloid scar. To try to control collagen production to prevent the recurrence of keloids, you may be given steroid injections and radiation, perhaps together.

Keloid recurrence is high, so for such surgery to be a success, it is essential for you to complete therapy as prescribed. If three radiation treatments are advised, be certain to have three; if weekly steroid injections are prescribed, be sure to keep all the appointments.

Be prepared for an initial healing phase of red, often raised, generally ugly tissue, which may well be more unsightly than the original scar. Persevere, however, as the healing may take two to four months, depending on your particular type of healing.

Do be prepared for this waiting period! Put away your mirror; postpone the final evaluation for at least four months and preferably six months; keep in mind how beautiful you are going to look; and, if possible, visit a spa midway in your recovery.

AESTHETIC SURGERY

Contour Surgery

To facilitate their reading of a face, portrait artists sketch it by dividing it into equal halves, thirds, or quarters, depending on their view. This is made possible because there is a measure of geometric harmony in the face, and if there is a major distortion (for the face is rarely balanced), nature has a way of compensating. This compensation often creates feature weaknesses—thus the need for contour surgery on the nose, ears, chin, jaw, or lips.

Nose . . . the Most Favored of All Body Features

I've seen many bad nose jobs, probably because people didn't stop to think what a nose would look like had it been born right! Since it is so prominent, the nose is the most common site for contour surgery.

In blacks, the nasal bridge may be underdeveloped, resulting in wide, low bones and a nose with a flattened tip and flared nostrils —most of these can be altered surgically.

Your nose surgery. During your consultation the plastic surgeon will: go over the areas that need improvement and explain the technique to be used; perhaps use an artist or photographer to illustrate the change planned; solicit your input and include it in your "re-look" plan if practical.

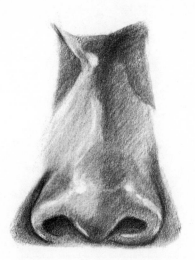

Surgery of this kind is performed in the hospital or in a private clinic, usually under local anesthesia with heavy sedation.

To build up your nasal bridge, the surgeon will use a silicone implant, your own bone, or your own cartilage. All three will do the job, and each has different advantages.

A cast may be applied for about a week. It can be dyed to match your skin tone . . . and in case you're wondering, autographed nose casts are definitely OUT! ✓

The nasal tissues may remain swollen for several months. Once again, you must have patience, for the final result cannot be judged for at least six months.

Reduce Protruding Ears

Thanks to the page-boy hair style, overly prominent or excessively large ears could long be hidden away. But . . . there is another way: They can also be contoured into more normal alignment and size.

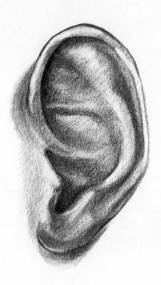

The most common ear disfigurements are protruding, or "Dumbo," ears and too large ears.

Protruding ears can be easily repositioned closer to the head, leaving a relatively inconspicuous scar on the back side of the ear. This is done, under local or general anesthesia, by removing skin behind the ear to expose the enlarged cartilage. The excessive part is weakened or removed; the ear is then folded and fixed into a more favorable position with sutures behind the ear. Anyone with a keloid tendency should approach this operation with caution.

Overly large ears can be reduced in size, but a scar will be visible. This is done by removing tissue from the upper ear. Where the wound ends are joined, there is a visible scar on the upper surface of the ear.

The recovery period from ear surgery is brief. A protective dressing usually is worn for three to five days followed by an elastic bandage or protective scarf worn while sleeping for an additional week.

The Chin . . . Be It Not Double or Weak

Weakness of the chin muscles, which will lead to a double chin, does not occur commonly in blacks; nevertheless, it does occur. Often it is associated with an ill-defined neck angle and a short neck.

Today's man has the option of altering his chin contour by growing hair. But women and men who wish to be clean-shaven have the option of chin implants or chin-plasty (see discussion on chin-plasty below, in section on surgery of aging) to achieve their desired face shape.

A chin implant results in a stronger, more prominent facial profile. In this procedure, silicone rubber is inserted either through the mouth or from an incision under the chin to create a pocket over the chin. The implant is carved for aesthetic balance and seated in place.

After surgery, the chin remains swollen for six to eight months.

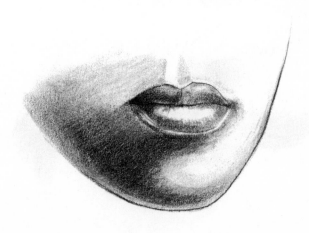

Ice packs followed by warm compresses are good for circulation during this time.

Patience is essential. It will take several months for the final results to be appreciated.

Jaw Line . . . Don't Let It Be a Breaker

The lower jaw can be excessively small or, more commonly in people with dark skins, it can be excessively large.

Bimaxillary protrusion, or monkey-shaped mouths. A common combination in blacks is a too-forward jaw position (bimaxillary protrusion) of the front segment of both jaws, which imparts a fullness to both the upper and lower lip areas. This contour disharmony may be considered disfiguring. It can be altered in a major surgical procedure.

In altering this contour, the surgeon fractures the jaw, then repositions it into a more balanced, functional, and aesthetic alignment. Usually the teeth are wired together for six to eight weeks while the bone heals.

Since this necessitates a light or blenderized diet, it's a good time to lose weight . . . and it's a good time for writing since you can't do much talking.

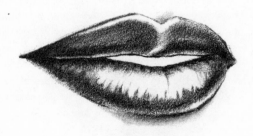

Another jaw condition is referred to as "mandibular prog-nathism," when the lower jaw is too prominent and the lower front teeth extend in front of the upper teeth.

Before any alteration of this is done (the procedure is similar to that just described), clinical examination, dental X-rays and medi-cal reconstruction photographs are required.

Lovable Lips

Excess size—hypertrophy—of one or both lips is not uncommon in persons with dark skins. It is characterized by fullness of the ex-ternal lip, of the underlying mucosa, and even of the muscles.

Surgery to reduce the lips is relatively minor. An incision is made inside the mouth, tissue removed, and sutures placed. Swelling can be significant, but the sutures are removed in about a week. The resulting scar is inconspicuous.

Surgery for Acne

Scarring following acne is less common in the black than in the Caucasian. Indeed, acne itself is less frequent and less severe in blacks. It occurs, nevertheless, and in some blacks, it is of significant magnitude and concern to need treatment.

First principle. Defer surgery until the acne is in a "burned-out" phase.

Second principle. Acne surgery, or dermabrasion, is designed to smooth an uneven surface. It is analogous to refinishing a scratched antique table. The more shallow the scratches, the better the result. Saucer-shaped shallow scars can be improved more than deeper pits. The surgeon, unlike the refinisher, can only remove so many layers of skin. One must leave the deeper layers to provide the re-generative elements for new skin.

Third principle. Pigmentation is a problem for the black patient considering dermabrasion. If the pigment cells are penetrated in an effort to minimize scarring, there may be significant pigment loss.

A test area out of sight, as on the hairline or just in front of the ear, can be used to evaluate the pigment changes. The surgical technique and postoperative treatment are used in the test area. If, after six to ten weeks, the pigment changes are acceptable, a full-face dermabrasion can be scheduled.

In dermabrasion, success is attained through diligent planing and replaning of uneven scars with mechanical instruments. The treatment area is a anesthetized before dermabrasion. Dermabrasion requires great skill, in that the scars must be removed while the hair follicles and glands are preserved to ensure regeneration of new tissue.

Postoperatively, it is up to the surgeon whether the area is bandaged or left open to dry. Major dermabrasion renders you homebound (or spa-bound) for eight to ten days while healing takes place.

Thereafter, the skin stays red and requires makeup for color harmony for three to four months while normal skin color is restored.

Convalescence from dermabrasion is longer and more involved than for most other cosmetic facial surgery.

Surgery of Aging

Operations to reduce facial age changes are particularly successful in the black male or female with no unusual scarring problems. The reason for this success is their relative absence of facial and eyelid wrinkles. While facelifts, chin-plasty, and eyelid-plasty are quite successful at removing loose hanging skin, they are weak at removing wrinkles, crow's feet, and etched lines at the corners of the eyelids.

Facelifts

The facelift can best minimize age changes in the neck and jowl area. Good candidates are men and women over forty who have hanging skin on the lower two thirds of the face and neck and who are at their lowest comfortable weight.

It will take about six weeks for you to see and enjoy the "new you" following a facelift. It is done under local or general anesthesia in a hospital or private clinic.

Incisions begin in the temple area, go down the hairline, and end behind the ear in the back scalp area. (Afterwards is a good time for your new hair style.) Through these incisions, one of the bands

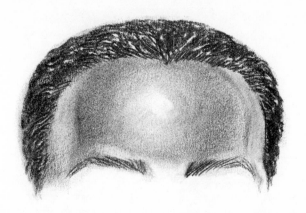

of facial muscles is tightened to effect the "lift." The skin is then redraped, the excess skin is removed, and the wound is sutured.

Often dressings are used for twenty-four to forty-eight hours. Bruising and swelling generally persist for ten to fourteen days but may last longer. Numbness and tightness are common complaints.

What a perfect time to go to a spa where you can get your spirits lifted too and remain to recuperate!

Chin-plasty

Chin-plasty is a small but effective procedure used to minimize an early "turkey gobbler" chin. Generally it is done under local anesthesia in a private clinic. An incision is made along a prominent fold or wrinkle line under the chin. Loose skin, excess fat, and some muscle are removed; and the skin is tightened and sutured.

The sutures are removed in about a week and healing is complete (the scar hidden away under the chin) in six to ten weeks' time.

Eyelid-plasty

The eyelid operation removes loose hanging skin from the upper

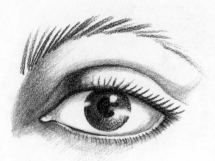

eyelids, "fat bags" from the lower eyelids, or picks up the corner of the eyelids to open the eyes more widely.

It is done under local or general anesthesia in the private clinic or hospital. Although it requires meticulous work (the operation may take up to two hours), it is not debilitating.

The eyelids may be bruised and swollen for a few days, but the discomfort is minimal. Dark glasses for ten to fourteen days not only will hide the more telltale signs but also will add an aura of mystery and excitement.

If you aren't totally pleased with the way you look, by all means be good to yourself and enjoy the beauty cosmetic surgery can bring you.

6

Your Face:
The Shaving Grace

CLEANSING, protection, lubrication, and stimulation are the goals of corrective shaving. While most stout-hearted men take the subject of physical fitness very seriously, facial skin fitness and maintenance are subjects about which most know very little. This despite the billions of industrial dollars spent in developing fine cosmetics to help you in your shaving quest . . . Cosmetics? You would never dare!

But please *do* dare. Enlightened males realize that the correct application of a cosmetic before, during, and after a shave is absolutely necessary if you are to achieve the look you want to have—smooth, clean, soft-to-the-touch, inviting.

These tips on shaving and skin care I like to call "Basic Trumpet." The awe-inspiring sound of the trumpet has long been used as a symbol of power and wealth; and a well-shaved face is the same. Keeping your shave finely tuned and your complexion staccato and sharp as the trumpet involves using common sense and an arsenal of fine products.

But before we get into that, let's look at some historical notes on shaving. I can imagine the first shaving or plucking of hairs must have been done by strong cave-dwelling men having nothing much to do but test their strength by removing their own facial hairs.

Cave paintings from prehistoric days depict what may have been man's first shaving instruments—shells and sharpened flints. Although history records the razor in Rome as early as the sixth century B.C., shaving was considered an effeminate Greek behavior pattern and did not come into vogue for another 150 years or so. According to one account, Alexander the Great introduced shaving into Greece when he ordered his soldiers to be clean-shaven to avoid being seized by the beard by their enemies!

By the fourth century B.C., shaving had apparently gained respectability and status—razors from that date found in Egyptian tombs were made of copper or solid gold. Herodotus credited the Egyptians' intense love of cleanliness as the impetus for their shaving.

Shaving truly became a fine art in the eighteenth and nineteenth centuries in England with the introduction of steel razors crafted by the artisans of Sheffield. The next advances were in the United States with the introduction of the safety razor in 1895 and the electric shaver in the early 1930s.

THE FIRST STEP—EXAMINE YOUR FACE

To examine your face properly, you'll need a good light source and a mirror that magnifies and casts a true image. With a magnifying mirror you can get a good close-up look at your face, which is important for finding even the most minor flaws of which you should be aware when you shave. Place the mirror so its angle gives you an under-the-chin view and side views as well.

For the best results, have a three-day beard growth when you conduct your examination.

Don't be rushed when you examine your face . . . Relax . . . Have classical or some soft, calming, easy-listening music surrounding you as you study your face and decide how best to handle your facial hair. Don't rush yourself. Decide carefully. Do you wish to be clean-shaven or bearded? If bearded, what shape beard or mustache and what length?

And while the examination is going on, think about the special things you should remember about shaving and while you are shaving. And what you'll be looking for.

What to Look For

Look first at where your hair grows and how it grows—what direction, what pattern, etc. Note especially the sensitive areas for hair growth—above the lip, high on the cheeks near to the eye, on the neck.

Mustache hairs—the hairs above the lip—are just as sensitive as eyebrow hairs and should be shortened with scissors before they are shaved.

Those few hairs high on the cheeks under the eye should be removed with tweezers.

Be very careful when shaving the creases in the neck. Be sure the skin is stretched so it is not loose. Beginning shavers and mild-brown-complexioned shavers should never shave the neck.

Note what skin type and texture you have, to help you decide which shaving technique is the right one for you (see Chapter 4 to find out how to determine your skin type).

If your skin is dry, it should always be oiled before you shave. Use a razor-blade shaver rather than electric shaver.

If your skin is oily, you should always use astringent before your shave. A light mask before every shave is best to brace the skin whether you use a razor-blade shaver or an electric shaver. Your beard should also be powdered before an electric shave.

If your skin is normal, take your pick of any of the various techniques.

Look for unruly hairs—those hairs which seem to grow long, then curl. These should be removed with tweezers.

Look for ingrown hairs. Don't ever shave over ingrown hairs. They require a special treatment which I'll cover later on in this chapter.

Look for pimples and blackheads and be careful not to shave over them. Mark them with a repair paste on a cotton swab.

Look for any darkened areas on your face and neck. Prolonged, frequent shaving can cause dark spots and they need a rest! So don't shave the areas until the darkness goes away. Lemon-peel rubs before and after shaving are helpful in retoning.

Now you've examined your face. What items do you need for a

good shave and what steps should you take to prepare your face and beard to be shaved?

THE SECOND STEP—HAVE THE ITEMS YOU NEED

The Hardware

Scissors. A fine pair, with pointed tips, which are comfortable in your grasp.

Tweezers. A pair with pointed tips and a pair squared-off at the ends.

Brushes. COMPLEXION BRUSH. A nicely shaped badger-hair brush with which you can either dry-massage or scrub your face and beard. SHAVING BRUSH. Again, a badger-hair brush is preferred. Get one with a beautiful handle you like to look at and hold. A

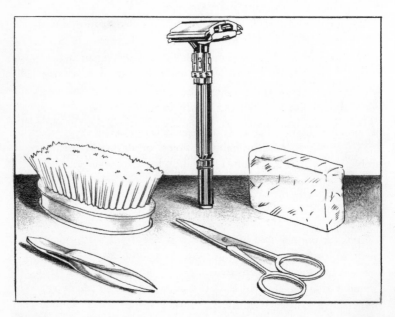

Shaving items. Left to right: Tweezers, brush, razor, scissors, alum block.

raccoon brush can be used, but the bristles tend to shed more easily than a badger-hair one.

Razor/shaver. The RAZOR I like is a double-edge Gillette adjustable safety razor. I prefer it for the weight of its handle and head. If you prefer another, choose one which feels comfortable in your hand and moves across your face well. SHAVER. I like the Remington electric shaver, which I consider to be the best balanced. Foreign-made shavers tend to have higher-quality workmanship, especially those made in West Germany.

Blades. Use fine double-edged stainless steel blades. You will get a closer, more gentle shave if you use the blade only once. However, never use the same blade more than two times.

Straight-edge razor. To be used in powder shaves only.

The Software

Shaving oil. A preshave solution for creating an oil base if you are going to use soap or cream for a razor shave.

Shaving cream, gel, or soap. The choice is a personal one. You may wish to alternate them.

CREAM. The most widely used cream is the aerosol variety. Of these, I like Rise Menthol. Cream should be fingered on and should always be moist. Apply only when you are ready to shave each area and remove immediately after application.

GEL. A gel has the value of being see-through and it is a favorite of so-called high yellows. It is especially valuable for protecting your skin when ingrown hairs, pimples, or darkened areas are a problem. A gel should not be allowed to dry before you shave.

SOAP. Shaving soap is used for that old-fashioned lather shave. A shaving soap should have a castile base with natural oil (olive oil is the most common). My own choice is the popular Williams Shaving Mug Soap.

Alum crystal block. An after-shave must, no matter what the technique, is an alum crystal block, to provide bracing for the pores and to stanch nicks or cuts (although you shouldn't get these, if your shaving equipment is balanced). Moisten it with water or toning astringent before applying it to your face.

After-shave astringent. Any mild astringent will do, such as witch hazel mixed with cornflower water or any mild after-shave to give

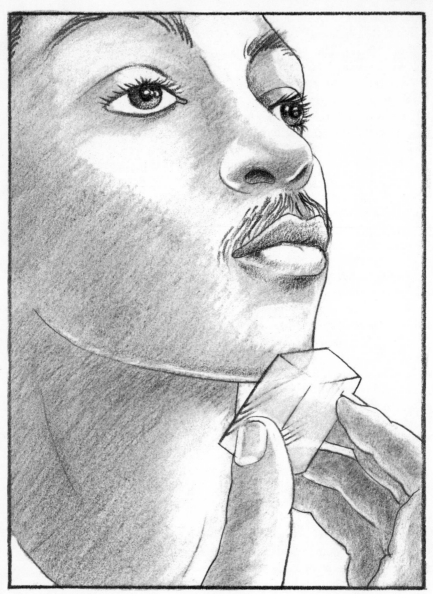

Use an alum crystal block after all types of shaving.

your skin a smarting, fresh feeling. For sensitive skin, a blemish astringent is preferable.

Mask. A quick-drying mask should be used three times a week following your shave. The mask can be rinsed off in the shower. Use any of the masks in Chapter 2.

Moisturizers or softening cream. A light cream or lotion will protect the natural moisture of your skin. Use a surface, not a penetrating lotion.

THE THIRD STEP—THE SHAVE ITSELF

Shaving brush, cup, and soap . . . the last American coat of arms, now gone away. Yet you can still get a good razor shave from a barber today, and that is an excellent way for you to learn how to shave correctly and how to solve any shaving problems you have. (But wherever did the shoeshine boy go?)

The Preshave Ritual

Before you even think about shaving, your beard should be at least a $\frac{1}{16}$-inch hair growth, long enough to permit your fingertip to feel the growth when you rub your face. And, very important, your face should be thoroughly cleansed, toned, and stimulated before you shave.

Cleansing and Toning

Use a complexion brush and soap to cleanse your face. Then rinse. Pat dry with a cotton square or washcloth presoaked with toning astringent. Use 5″ × 5″ thin cotton washcloths soaked in a metal pan of water as your hot towels.

Stimulating

Briskly pat your face both before and after shaving to stimulate your skin and hair. Or dry-massage your face with a brush.

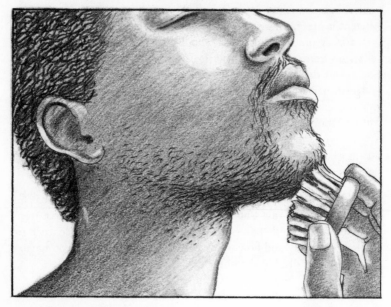

Brush facial hair with warm soap and water before shaving.

Now the Shave

To get a good, close shave you must make lots of different faces while you are shaving so as to have a flat, tight skin surface. There should be no hard reaching for places. Shave a section at a time. Get a close-up look in a mirror. Angle your mirror for side views and under-the-chin view.

When in doubt about shaving a particular area, don't; use scissors or tweezers instead. Remove coarse-textured hairs and hard-to-get-at hairs with sharp pointed scissors and pointed tweezers.

Most important to insure a good long-lasting shave is the proper moisture. With each shave, a peeling of the epidermis and loss of moisture occur. Proper moisture not only softens the skin before shaving to make hair removal easier, but also protects the skin after shaving.

For the Electric Shave

After cleansing, toning, and brushing dry, brush on a thin layer of natural dust talc. Use shaver to remove beard. Pat on mild astringent.

For the Razor-Blade Shave

Apply shaving cream or gel thinly enough so that you can still see the hairs to be shaved.

Shave your face carefully a section at a time, taking care to shave with the direction of your hair growth, not against it. Use fast, quick strokes.

When you have finished removing the hair, apply an after-shave freshener and briskly pat it dry with a washcloth.

Apply your alum block.

IF YOU DECIDE TO BE BEARDED

If you decide to be bearded, go to a professional barber, a makeup artist, or a facial salon for assistance in designing your beard to be the length and shape you want.

Beards can be corrective. They can hide a facial flaw—they can strengthen a weak chin, they can make a face appear fuller. Or they can just add distinction and class.

For a special occasion, you may even want to have your beard tinted. For this, go to a professional. Do not do it yourself!

And the best thing about a beard is that you can simply shave it away if you don't like it or if you tire of it.

REMOVAL OF INGROWN HAIRS

Basically there are two types of ingrown hairs—long ingrown hairs which are usually on the neck and short ingrown hairs which can be on the face as well as on the neck.

This condition occurs frequently if you have coarse and curly facial hair. It may also be caused by incorrect shaving that goes

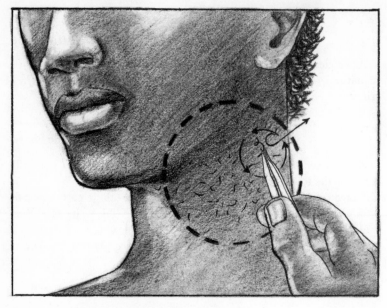

Remove any ingrown hairs before shaving.

against the grain of hair growth as well as by natural changes in skin texture over the years.

Remove ingrown hairs as the illustration shows. Locate the hair using a good light source and a magnifying mirror. Pull on the hair a little bit with pointed tweezers. Then manipulate the hair gently, rocking it back and forth in its inflamed cradle until it is freed and can be removed.

A FEW SPECIAL NOTES

Use softening creams and healing camphor creams at night to prepare for a morning shave.

Take a shaving rest when you vacation, especially if you shave more than three times a week.

If you have a light beard growth, shave at night to avoid that "just-shaved" look in the daytime.

7

Keeping Your Body Fit

YOUR DIET, your feelings, and your general health are the internal forces that affect your skin. If you want to be beautiful outside, you must first be beautiful inside. Your body is your temple, and it is your responsibility to ensure its sanctity.

Transforming the inner you into truth and beauty requires you to consider the following.

• Diet
• Exercise
• Rest

DIET

Our prehistoric predecessors were smarter than we are. Contrary to the image of Fred Flintstone gnashing his teeth and gorging on a dinosaur leg is the scientific evidence of at least a million and a half years of herbivores in our past ancestry.

Only relatively recently have human diets contained animal products, and they are certainly not helping human health problems. With such diets, you must seek to insure the healthy functioning of the endocrine glands, to stimulate cell metabolism, and to promote the optimum formation and transport of healthy blood—your nurturer!

This job will be a lot easier for you if you understand what your body needs and doesn't need to do its job. You need water, protein, fats, carbohydrates, fiber, at least fourteen vitamins, and more than twenty minerals and essential trace metals!

Since this isn't a nutrition book and I'm not a nutritionist, I won't delve into those here. If you think you have a diet problem, you can see a clinical nutritionist who will be able to analyze any diet deficiencies or excesses through dietary intake assessment, hair analysis for minerals, and blood analysis for vitamins. Then, if you need to take supplements, you will know exactly which ones and what amount you should take.

Golden Rules

I will offer a few golden rules to help your blood flow freely to nourish the outer as well as the inner you.

Reduce your intake of salt and refined sugars. Season your food with herbs and spices instead. You'll get their benefits as well as reduce the ill-effects of the bad Ss. And you'll be delightfully surprised by the variety of taste sensations your palate enjoys, hitherto concealed by the bad Ss.

Eat less red meat. You may find that you'll have more energy and need less sleep.

Don't eat so many animal fats. Use margarine instead of butter and lard. Learn to eat things broiled or poached instead of fried.

Eat foods with high fiber content such as whole grains, fruits with their skins, and vegetables like cabbage.

Eat more raw fruits and vegetables. If you cook vegetables, steam them so their nutrients remain.

Cut down on caffeine—on coffee, tea, and cola drinks. Drink fruit juices, herbal brews, and mineral water instead.

Bypass the candy store and go to the fruit stand instead. An apple a day keeps more than the doctor away.

The Miracle Workings of Garlic

Wrapped tear drops of wonder, garlic is indeed a miracle vegetable. It can be used externally, directly on a pimple; it is used by many internally as a digestive.

The nutritional key to beauty lies in a sound digestion and garlic is a digestive wonder. Its use for this purpose is particularly common in Japan. Garlic may have come to Japan from China through Korea, along with Buddhism, in the early Christian era. So powerful is it seen as a medicinal stimulant that, even today, there are some Zen temples which prohibit garlic on their premises, along with four other strong vegetables—onion, leek, scallion, and ginger.

Although some find its smell repugnant, its value as a digestive may make the smell worth enduring. When you've overeaten, take two garlic-oil capsules and see how much better you feel.

And Now for Mama's Periodic Cures

When I was a little boy and right on through my growing-up years, at the end of every summer and after all the feasting holidays, my sisters and I got therapeutic doses of castor oil to purge our systems and get us ready for a clean, new start back to school.

I believe in this "cure" just as my mother does. For me, a periodic "purging" is essential to the healthy functioning of my metabolism and for a healthy outer glow.

Mama's other cure, a dose of Sal Hepatica, helped two of my five sisters feel fewer of the premenstrual symptoms and to control those time-of-the-month pimples.

When You Need to Shed

Shedding pounds is both a science and an art—its theory is science and its practice is art! There are hundreds of diets you can choose from, weight-loss programs galore, and so-called fat farms to escape to if you're rich enough and just can't, or don't, want to do it on your own.

Whichever way you go . . . if you have more than a few pounds to lose or if you have a medical problem, you should ALWAYS GET THE ADVICE AND COUNSEL OF A PHYSICIAN before you begin dieting.

No one ever claimed that dieting is easy . . . but it is usually well worth the effort. And here are a few points to bear in mind:

You may be too fat because you have bad eating habits that you must change to be thin. <u>*You* must want to lose weight, not diet because someone else wants you to.</u> Start doing other things when you feel like eating to distract you from food. Stop thinking you should eat every time you feel like it. Above all else, keep in your mind how beautiful the new, thinner you will be. Convince yourself you like apples more than doughnuts, carrot sticks more than potato chips . . . and so on . . . and so on . . . and so on.

Here are several diets I think sound special and include foods to make you beautiful as well. Don't try to stay on any of them for longer than a week. And remember . . . SEE A PHYSICIAN BEFORE YOU DIET!

The Waldorf 600 Diet

Make the following beautiful salad. You can eat it 4 times a day and still have only about 600 calories. But don't eat anything else.

	Calories
¼ head lettuce	17
½ sliced tomato	15
½ green pepper	5
1 carrot	21
½ cup sliced fresh mushrooms	15
½ chopped apple	35
2 teaspoons diet mayonnaise	40
¼ sliced zucchini	6
¼ sliced cucumber	6
TOTAL	160

If you don't want to eat the entire salad 4 times a day, select only the things you want. Just don't take over 650 calories a day!

The Good-Skin Diet

This diet gives your skin a boost and helps you shed pounds quickly. It is beneficial for persons who have acne.

Eat 3 times a day to satisfy yourself, but not in excess. Eat a lot of lean meat—poultry without skin, lean cuts of beef, lean fish, and shell fish. Eat fresh fruits and unseasoned vegetables in moderation. Drink at least 6 big glasses of water a day. Don't eat any fats—no butter, margarine, milk, cream, sugar, or cheese or any products made with any of these. Don't eat highly seasoned foods or pizza. Drink nothing alcoholic.

Banana-Milky Way Diet

This diet *requires* medical supervision and supplemental nutrients.

4 bananas
3 8-ounce glasses of skimmed milk
1 8-ounce glass of water with each banana and each glass of milk

While you're on this diet, you can also mix up a little It's Bananas Eye Cream (see recipe on p. 36). Just don't forget and eat the honey—it goes in the cream, not your mouth!

Edgar Cayce Apple Diet

The teachings of the psychic Edgar Cayce offer his insights into health. He was convinced of the value of an almond a day—"For the almond blossomed when everything else died. Remember this is life."

I've always enjoyed his raw-apple diet, to cleanse the system. The diet prescribes 3 days of raw apples only, preceded by a spoonful of olive oil, to eliminate toxic forces from the system. Try different varieties of apples—for example, Arkansas Black for breakfast; Granny Smith for lunch; Oregon Red in the evening; and Delicious, either red or gold, for that in-between delight! And take one tablespoon Greek olive oil every morning.

Fasting

Obviously, the total fast is the quickest way to lose weight. For it, you should have clearance from your physician as well as his or her supervision and advice on how many days to fast. You must drink at least eight 8-ounce glasses of water every day you fast.

Remember that you will not have a lot of energy when you fast. Only fast during periods when stresses—climatic, environmental, emotional, and medical—are low. Supplements—vitamins, minerals, etc.—will be necessary.

EXERCISE

The ancient Greek physician Hippocrates, called the father of medicine, said, "That which is used develops. That which is not wastes away." So it is with our bodies. Our technological advances have encouraged us to be sedentary, since we aren't often called on for muscle power.

So, one in five of us has back problems, and as we age, we may become rigid and tired, lose our suppleness, agility, the beauty of fluid motion. How sad, since it is so unnecessary.

Exercise improves our general well-being. It increases circulation and, in so doing, helps our skin to flourish.

Exercise is available to all of us—it can range from the simple and inexpensive to the rigorous and costly. Choose the exercise program that best suits your moods, your likes, your lifestyle, and your budget. If you're not sure what is best for you, the Ys—YMCA, YWCA, and YM/YWCA—can give you advice (they also have exercise classes at nominal fees). My own recommendations are the following:

Brisk walking. Many New Yorkers stay in very good shape because they walk far and fast to go up and down many subway steps. It may not always be scenic, but you can't beat New York City for walking exercise.

Jogging and running. One of our latest crazes—and a good one —is jogging. If you jog, think beautiful thoughts the whole time. Be sure to have good shoes to avoid ankle and leg injuries. What jogger doesn't have a little thought somewhere inside about training for the Boston marathon? Running takes discipline and endurance. If you have an abundance of both, running may be right for you.

Dancing. Dancing can be an aesthetic, sophisticated approach to exercise. It can give you grace, poise, and beauty along with a workout. Choose the type of dancing that suits you—be it classical ballet, jazz, aerobic, psychocalisthenic, or tap dancing.

Cycling. In addition to its exercise value, cycling gives you a great way to get around town.

Tennis, squash, racquetball. All three are sophisticated sports for the harried business executive who loves competition.

Seasonal outdoor exercising. For the outdoor person, nothing can beat seasonal outdoor sports. For variety and a seasonal approach, try hiking and backpacking in the fall; volleyball and softball in the spring; water-skiing and sailing in summer; cross-country or down-hill skiing and snowshoeing in the winter.

No matter which exercise or exercises you decide upon, the key to their benefits is in doing them regularly. If you hate exercise, have a weekly massage, followed by a good hot steaming.

REST

You cannot attain a sense of well-being through diet and exercise alone. Your inner light, your spirit, must have some restful times in order to send forth glowing rays of beauty to the outer you . . . to make your skin lovelier. "Except the Lord build the house, they labor in vain that build it." (Psalms 127)

Meditation

Meditation stills the mind, takes the consciousness to higher levels, and places the person who is meditating in a state of gentle alertness. It frees the mind from daily cares and allows positive energies to flow throughout the body.

You don't have to trek to Tibet or take a course to learn how to meditate. Your own home can be your ashram. Here's what you do.

Select a regular place and time of day to meditate for 15 to 30 minutes. Sit or kneel in a comfortable position. Gently tap the top of your head three times to beckon your soul. Be very still and let your mind go free—seek emptiness which is wholeness. If you cannot, select a spiritual word that is special to you and chant it aloud or silently . . . slowly . . . and over and over again. Feel in unity with everything else—with all life, with time . . . the cosmic oneness.

Music

"Music is a moral law. It gives a soul to the universe, wings to the mind, flight to the imagination, a charm to sadness, gaiety and life to everything. It is the essence of order and leads to all that is good and just and beautiful."—PLATO, *The Republic*, Bk. III.

Music has been used therapeutically for ages—in the Bible, David chased away Saul's devils with his harp. And it leads, just as Plato said, to beauty. And do leave those glorious heavy beats at the disco! A beauty treatment requires gentle sound—Beethoven, Mozart, Brahms . . .

PONDERING BLESSINGS ON BEAUTY

Makeup artist Way Bandy has this to say of health, beauty, and spirit: "In the sixties people looked at their spirits. In the seventies people looked at their health and bodies. It is my hope that in the eighties, people will finally acknowledge that cooperation with nature on all levels is the only way that we can have the good life that we want."

8

Cosmetics:
Simplicity to Complexity

WALK UP to the cosmetic counter in a department store or in a drugstore or go into one of those fabulous, luxurious little cosmetics boutiques and what do you see? . . . A rich, eye-catching, and often confusing array of beautifully packaged, glamorously presented products to choose from. You will be helped by a demure young lady who, you hope, has some training in skin care . . . and she will urge you on to try the latest wonder cream and show you how it looks under a lamp scientifically designed to flatter you, her, and the product.

It's a wonderful luxury trip, one I think everyone should indulge in when spirits are low and need a lift! Just sitting there trying beautiful products in such a flattering light surrounded by pleasant fragrances is enough to make one feel wonderful.

But before I go any further, let me clearly separate two categories of cosmetics. First, there are those used in basic and special skin care, which we have discussed up to now in this book. This category includes—

• Cleansers and soaps
• Fresheners
• Toners
• Astringents

- Moisturizers
- Eye creams
- Night creams
- Skin lotions
- Facial masks

The other category of cosmetics are applied purely for ornament —in other words, makeup products. Included are—

- Base or foundation makeup
- Cover sticks
- Rouges and blushers
- Powders
- Eyebrow pencils and sticks
- Eyeliners
- Eye shadow
- Mascara
- Eyelashes
- Lip colors
- Nail enamels
- Hair-care products including shampoos, rinses, conditioners, sprays, straighteners, color rinses, thickeners, and restorers
- Antiperspirants and deodorants
- Perfumes, colognes, fragrant waters

If you use makeup, be sure that you are using it to enhance your natural beauty, not to conceal some condition that can be corrected with proper skin care. Sadly, before dark-skinned people were reminded of skin care by those who knew, many of them preferred to put on makeup to cover up a problem than to take the trouble and discipline themselves to follow a careful daily routine that would help correct it. We have come a long way since light and dark Egyptian and nut brown.

MAKEUP

For Your Face

Remember that the essence of makeup is highlighting and coloring, not covering. Your delicate tissues can't handle much weight and must breathe . . . so use only one layer on any one place.

Don't use foundation on areas you will apply darker colors to. If you do, you will be coloring your foundation, not your face. Select a foundation light in texture, in a water base rather than an oil base. To determine the ideal one for you, try it out on your neck—this is the area most like your face and the area you will want your foundation to blend into.

Spread it on sparingly!

Choose your makeup carefully—one that feels good to you and you feel good about. If you find a particular brand of cosmetics that gives you good results, stick with it . . . unless you're adventurous. If so, then by all means experiment, and often.

Use as many natural products as possible without chemicals or preservatives. These are most easily purchased at natural food stores.

For Your Eyes

Understated, natural, and elegant eye makeup can enhance the beauty of your eyes and draw attention to your well-cared-for complexion. Eye makeup requires special attention, as follows . . .

Instead of foundation cream, which you should not use under your eye makeup, use the following recipe for your very own eye foundation. (This mixture is good for your entire face as well as for your eye area.)

2 drops light-textured liquid foundation
1 drop light-textured moisturizer
3 drops mineral water

• Using a clean, empty eye dropper, place ingredients on a small dish.
• Mix them into a smooth cream with your fingertip.

About the liquid foundation. Select a liquid foundation, light-textured, with water rather than oil base. Choose a color to match the skin of your neck so that, when you blend it downward, you won't have a line of demarcation. Your neck is the place to test for color, as noted above.

About the moisturizer. Select a light-textured cream moisturizer, one that will lubricate as well as moisturize.

About the mineral water. Select any commercial bottled mineral water.

Daytime Eyes

Step 1. With a touching, pressing, patting movement, delicately blend in the above mixture onto your entire eye area—over, under, and on the eyelid itself. Treat your eye like an eggshell you don't want to break.

Step 2. Using the same liquid foundation you used in the above mixture, with a cotton swab, place a dot of foundation on the eye areas that tend to be dark: (1) the little valley or structural indentation under your eyes by your nose; (2) the outside corners beside your eyes; and (3) the hollow inside corner above your eyes under the orbital bones. Touch the foundation to blend and slightly lighten it so as not to make the skin look coated or like crepe.

Step 3. Using another light-textured liquid foundation several shades darker than the skin of your neck (always neutral beige, not with a red or yellow quality), place one dot on each eyelid. Blend the dots with the fingertip-touch technique over your entire upper lid areas from eyelashes to eyebrows. The idea here is to make your eyes themselves more important by darkening the protruding areas so that they appear to recede while your eyes come out.

Step 4. Using a third light-textured liquid foundation several shades darker than the second (still neutral beige), put another dot on each eyelid directly above your lashes. Blend the dots with the touch technique on the lids directly over the eyeballs—not in the creases or on the orbital bones.

Step 5. With a black eyeliner pencil you have warmed and softened with your fingertips, lift each upper eyelid so you can see the pink rim. Using several sketchy movements, draw a line from the inside corner all the way to the outside corner. Release the eyelid. This line defines the shape of your eyes without the eyeliner actually showing.

Step 6. Using an eyelash curler, curl your top eyelashes and apply mascara while still curling top eyelashes.

Step 7. Apply waterproof black mascara to your top and bottom eyelashes. Remember as you apply mascara that you're coloring

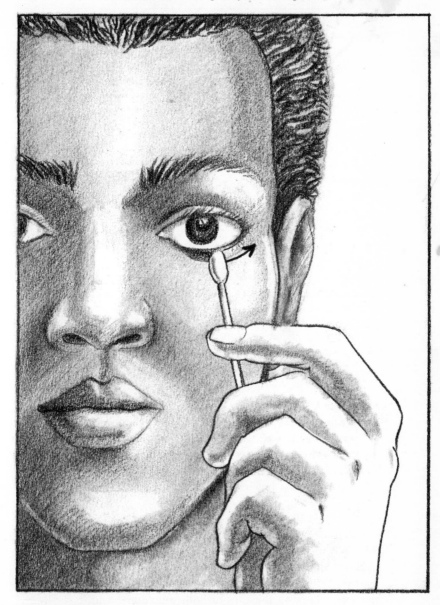

Apply foundation to dark areas under eyes.

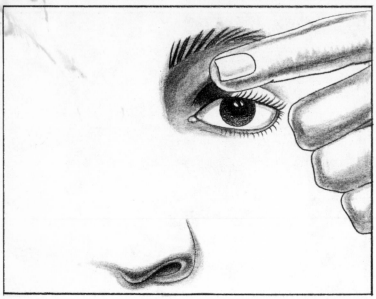

Darken your eyelids with color. Use brown or gray and apply with your fingertip, working from the corner of your eyes from nose to ear, for the best result.

each individual lash darker—don't put on too heavy a coating, which would cause lashes to stick together.

Step 8. With a dark gray or brown eyeliner pencil, delicately put several little dots along your lower eyelids, from the outside to the inside, just under your eyelashes. End where the eyelashes end, not beyond. With your fingertip blend the dots into a shadow effect.

Evening Eyes

For more dramatic evening eyes, begin by repeating Steps 1 through 5 as you would for daytime eyes.

Now follow the next six steps to finish your Evening Eyes!

Step 1. Using a black eyeliner pencil, softened with your fingertips, draw lines on the rims or both your upper and lower lids, all the way from the inside to the outside corners of your eyes. Make the lines intense and bold since the lines will gradually fade away.

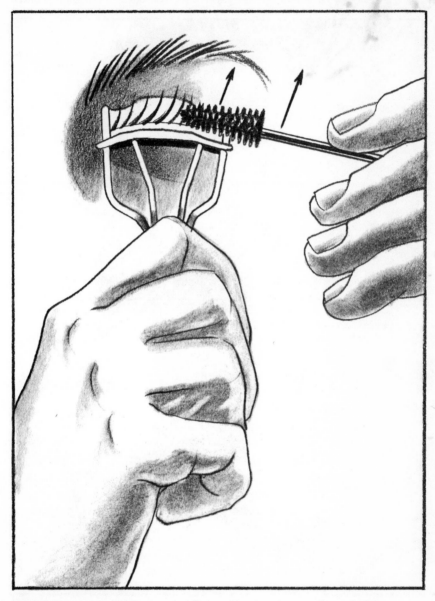

Apply mascara to eyelashes, holding curler in place to keep lashes apart.

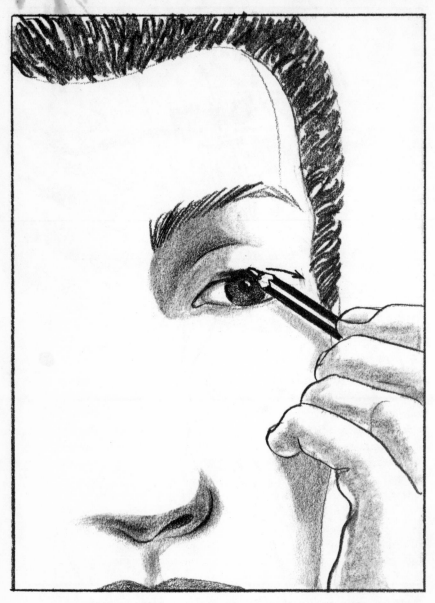

Draw a line directly over your top eyelashes with brown or gray eyeliner pencil.

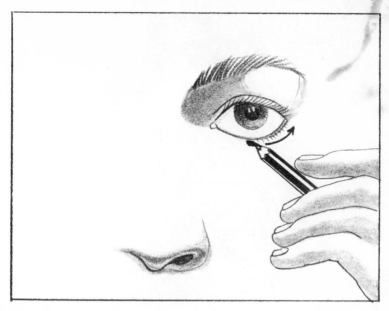

Draw a line under your eye too.

Step 2. With the same black eyeliner pencil, draw lines directly over your top eyelashes, from the inside to the outside corners. Use your fingertip to smudge and blend these lines for a shadow effect.

Step 3. Using a brown or gray eyeliner pencil, draw lines directly under your lower eyelashes from the inside to the outside corner. With your fingertip, smudge and blend these lines for a shadow effect.

Step 4. Using an eyelash curler, curl your top eyelashes.

Step 5. Use more mascara on both top and bottom eyelashes. Remember you want to create a darkening of each lash, not a mascara coating.

Step 6. Brush eyebrows upward, following the curve of the browline.

When you have mastered the basic tools and techniques for beautiful eyes as well as the use of standard colors, you can do the same

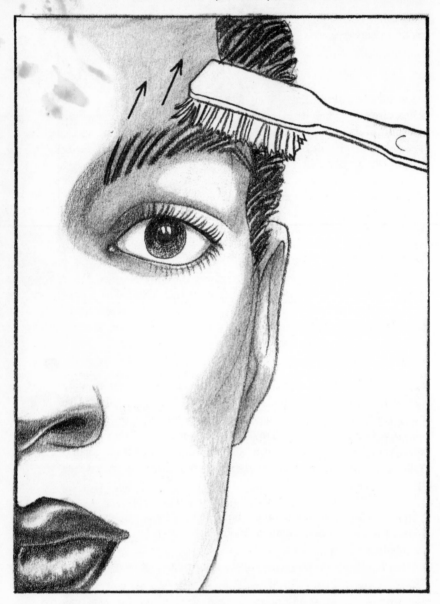

Brush your eyebrows upward for a finishing touch.

using other colors. Grays and browns are best, however, for sharp, bright, intense strong eye beauty.

For Your Hair

Specifically with regard to men . . .

Beautiful skin cannot be enjoyed and admired if it is not capped by beautiful hair. In appearance many say that hair is the crowning glory. Yet it is a crowning glory only if it is well kept. And to be well kept it must be easy to groom.

Until the 1960s, the hair styling of dark-skinned American men followed only one tradition—greased down and waxed "naturals," or "stocking caps" . . . these were the styles of our fathers and grandfathers too. This gave way to the freedom of the "Afro" about a decade ago—when people protested, "I won't get a process."

The hair of black men, having gone through this period of change, is searching for a new tradition in the 1980s with a textured look brought on by the quest for a softer "black-is-beautiful" image. So now we have the weak hair-relaxer perm aimed at softening the look and making combing and restyling easier.

A man's crowning glory these days demands three things—control; manageability; style. A hair tonic/lotion alternated with a spray-on brilliantine are important for hair styling. Tonics relieve oily or dry scalps, dandruff, and sometimes falling hair if its cause is clogged sebaceous glands or hair follicles, dehydration of the scalp, poor circulation, or infection.

Hair conditioning should be a regular part of a visit to your hairdresser. But before you go, to assist both you and your hairdresser in the renaissance of your hair, I suggest an application of some rich conditioner anywhere from five hours before right up to when you leave for your salon visit. My own choice is Hy Note, an avocado-pulp conditioner blended with essential oils; I find it is a wonderful conditioner for chemically treated hair or for anything else that has changed the texture of my hair.

If you're on a budget or if you love to experiment, try making your own avocado conditioner. To do this, blend an overripe avocado (one which has been on your window sill for at least a week and has turned black) with wheat-germ oil and vitamin E oil.

Massage in your conditioner, then wrap your hair in a plastic cap, and leave on as directed. Rinse out conditioner with lukewarm to cool water.

. After rinsing out the conditioner, shampoo with *two* shampoos—a hair-repair shampoo and a grooming shampoo.

Shampoo first with a hair-repair shampoo—perhaps a blend containing pine tar, coconut oil, lecithin, and distilled water—to benefit both your hair and your scalp.

Shampoo next with a grooming shampoo made with olive oil and an emulsifying (stabilizing) agent such as triethanolamine.

Rinse your hair completely. Then set your hair for its normal styling.

The Scent or Scents for You

There are so many kinds of perfumes, colognes, and fragrant waters that you can make a scent for yourself for every moment. Remember above all else that scents don't discriminate between males and females. A beautiful scent for one sex is just as beautiful for the other.

Scents that bespeak the flavors of nature are very individual—as if, when you wear it, you blend it with your very own bouquet.

Our delight in the scent experience is not just an inexplicable, easily dismissed fad. It is a reflection of our animal nature, an end result of deeply felt physical attraction.

Choose your scent to suit you—to create a mood, to cast a spell. Never let it permeate; never let it hover. Instead, let it waft; let it linger lightly. And most of all, let it be identified with you!

9

Cosmetics and Skin Care Terms You Should Know

ACETATES   Acetic acid salts used in astringents and perfumes.

ACETONE   A colorless liquid derived by oxidation or fermentation used in nail-polish removers.

ACRYLIC MONOMER   A tough rubbery agent used in artificial nails.

ALCOHOL (ETHANOL)   A volatile liquid widely used in cosmetics as a solvent.

ALOE GEL   A greenish herbal substance touted for its medicinal value, especially as a burn remedy. Used in cosmetics, particularly sun-tanning preparations.

ALUMINUM ACETATE   A compound used in solution as an astringent and antiseptic.

ALUMINUM CHLORIDE   Salt used in antiperspirants to retard the flow of perspiration.

ALUMINUM SILICATE   A substance obtained from clay and added to face powder for its anticaking and coloring properties.

ANTIOXIDANT   An agent that inhibits oxidation, used in various products to prolong their life.

ASTRINGENT   A preparation, usually liquid, used to make the skin feel fresh and tight by balancing surface moisture.

AZO DYES   Dyes used to give hair a temporary color.

BALSAM OF PERU A liquid fragrance used in masks, perfumes, and cream rinses.

BARRIER AGENTS Certain ingredients (including earths, waxes, gums, certain stearates, and talc) in creams and lotions that protect them against water and detergents.

BICARBONATE OF SODA (SODIUM BICARBONATE) A white powdery substance used as an antacid and for skin reactions to burns and insect stings.

BISMUTH COMPOUNDS Used when a pearliness is desired in a cosmetic.

BLEMISH CREAM Drying, soothing night cream for troubled complexions. A treatment ointment for pimples, acne, and blackheads.

BLUSHER A rougelike powder, stick, or cream used to put color on the cheeks.

BROMOFLUORESCEINS A group of soluble certified dyes in the yellow range, used in lipsticks.

CALCIUM CARBONATE A chalklike absorbent added to talc to remove its shine.

CAMPHOR A preservative and cooling ingredient used in many emollient creams, eye lotions, and fresheners or applied directly on skin for enlarged pores after cleansing.

CANDELILLA WAX A natural wax obtained from the candelilla shrub. May be used in facial masks.

CARBON BLACK (LAMPBLACK) An inorganic pigment used in eye shadow, eyebrow pencils, and mascara.

CARMINE LAKE A pigment used in eye cosmetics for shades of red.

CETYL ALCOHOL A white, waxy solid with a faint odor used as an emulsifier and emollient in perfumes, face creams, lotions, and lipsticks.

CHAMOMILE A natural substance, obtained from a flower, used to enhance the luster of blond hair.

CHLORHEXIDINE A sterilizing agent used in liquids and in feminine-hygiene sprays.

CHLOROXYLENOL A germicide and fungicide contained in feminine-hygiene sprays.

CHROMIC OXIDE An inorganic pigment frequently used for green shades of eye shadow.

CLEANSER A compound used to remove makeup, dirt and environmental pollutant particles, and normal excretions from the surface of the skin from head to toe.

COAL-TAR DYES Dyes obtained from bituminous coal formerly widely used to make cosmetic colors. Cannot be used in eye products by law. *A possible carcinogen.* Avoid if possible.

COLD CREAM The therapeutic and cosmetic forerunner of all modern skin cleansing products.

COLLAGEN A fibrous protein that comprises most of the white fiber in the connective tissue of animals, including man, especially in skin, muscles, and tendons. Used as a base for face creams, lotions, and hairdressing preparations.

COLOGNE A toilet water with a medium-strength fragrance.

COLORING AGENTS Any dyes, pigments, or other substances that give color to cosmetics.

COLOR LAKES Insoluble organic pigments prepared by precipitating soluble colors with forms of aluminum, calcium, potassium, zirconium, barium, or strontium. Used in eye shadow and lipstick.

COSMETICS Substances defined by the FDA as any articles "to be rubbed, poured, sprinkled, or sprayed on, introduced into, or otherwise applied to the human body or any part thereof for cleansing, beautifying, promoting attractiveness, or altering the appearance."

COVER STICK (BLEMISH STICK) A makeup product used to mask minor blemishes, discolorations, or shadows.

D&C COLOR A synthetic dye that is permitted in certified batches to be used in drugs and cosmetics.

DEODORANT A product or ingredient used to prevent the growth of odor-causing microorganisms.

DIETHANOLAMINE A colorless, viscous, hygroscopic liquid used in fatty-acid soaps.

EMOLLIENT CREAM A preparation used to make the skin feel soft and smooth; to reduce chafing, dryness, or roughness; and possibly to help retard development of wrinkles.

EMULSIFIER An agent that assists in the suspension of one liquid within another liquid. Used in cleansing creams and lotions.

EOSIN A group of colors in the red range. Used in lipstick.

ETHANOLAMINE A colorless viscous liquid widely used in detergents and as an emulsifying agent. Also used as a preservative in permanent waves.

EXT D&C COLOR A synthetic dye that is permitted in certified batches for external use only in drugs and cosmetics. Not for use on the lips or mucous membranes.

EYE CREAMS Softening creams for skin in the eye areas.

EYE-MAKEUP REMOVER A solution, usually on pads, especially designed to remove eye makeup.

EYE SHADOW Inert pigments used on the eyelids to flatter the eyes.

FACIAL MASK A substance applied to the face to cleanse it thoroughly while firming, cooling, and tightening the skin.

FATTY ACID A saturated acid—lauric, myristic, stearic, etc.—mixed with glycerin to form a fat used in soaps, etc.

FD&C COLOR A synthetic dye that the federal Food, Drug, and Cosmetic Act of 1938 allows to be used in food, drugs, and cosmetics.

FLAVORING An essence added to food for taste. May be used in homemade astringents.

FORMALDEHYDE A preservative used in nail polish and nail hardeners. Also used in hairsprays. Highly toxic; causes cancer in rats. Avoid if possible.

FOUNDATION MAKEUP A compound used to cover the skin both for a smooth, healthy appearance and as a protection against the wind, cold, and environmental pollutants.

FRESHENER A clear liquid used to make the skin feel cool and refreshed.

GLYCERIN A clear, odorless, syrupy liquid with a sweet taste, soluble in water and alcohol. Widely used in many cosmetics as a solvent, emollient, and moisturizer.

GLYCEROL MONOSTEARATE A pure, white or cream-colored wax-like solid with a faint odor and fatty agreeable taste, used in cleansers and creams.

GUANINE A natural pearling agent obtained from the scales of certain fish, used in nail polish to give a pearly luster.

GUMS Natural or synthetic water-soluble thickeners used in a variety of cosmetics.

HAIR CONDITIONER   A product used to soften hair, add moisture, and undo damage from other products.

HENNA   A natural reddish hair dye and highlighter and body coloring agent used since ancient times.

HERB   A natural plant product with medicinal or aromatic properties, added to various cosmetics for protective and/or enhancing effects.

HORMONE   A secretion of the endocrine glands such as estrogen or progesterone, which, added to creams, is alleged by some to enhance a youthful appearance and retard aging.

HUMECTANT   A substance used in cosmetics as a moisturizing agent.

IRON OXIDE SIENNA   An inorganic pigment used in eye cosmetics for brown shades.

ISOPROPYL PALMITATE   A colorless liquid which acts as an emollient or emulsifier in lotions, creams, and similar cosmetic products.

KAOLIN   A clay derivative in powder form used in skin-covering agents to absorb the skin's oils.

LANOLIN   A purified fatty substance from the wool of sheep used in all categories of cosmetics. A natural emulsifier as well as an emollient, it is absorbable by the skin.

LECITHIN   A waxy solid that is a natural part of all animal nerve and brain tissue. Widely used as a food supplement.

LIP BRUSH   A small brush, usually of mink or sable hair, used to trace a sharp outline around the lips which is then filled in with lipstick.

LIP CREAM   A softening cream for the lips.

MASCARA   A compound put onto the eyelashes to make them longer, thicker, and more lustrous-looking.

MENTHOL   An aromatic alcohol-derived substance used in cosmetics to give the skin a cool feeling.

MYRISTYL ALCOHOL   A white solid, insoluble in water, used in ointments, shampoos, and specialty cleansing preparations.

NIGHT CREAM   A softening face cream specially formulated for use before sleeping.

OXIDIZER   A developing agent—peroxide is an example—used with oxidation-type hair dyes to achieve the desired color.

PARABENS   A term used in the cosmetics industry for certain benzene derivatives—for example, p-hydroxybenzoic acid, propyl paraben, butylparaben, and methylparaben—the most widely used preservatives and bacteria and fungus fighters. Found in most types of skin care and makeup products.

PARAFFIN   A tasteless, odorless waxy derivative of petroleum used in many cosmetics as a stiffener.

PERFUME (FRAGRANCE)   Any of the more than five thousand substances used to give a pleasant smell to a cosmetic product or used alone on the skin.

PEROXIDE   An oxidizing and bleaching agent used in hair-coloring products, skin bleaches, permanent waves, and cold creams. Specifically, hydrogen peroxide.

PETROLATUM (PETROLEUM JELLY)   An emollient derived from petroleum, used in many cosmetics and as a skin lubricant.

pH   A chemical symbol indicating the acid-alkaline ratio of a solution. Measured on a scale of 1 to 14 with pH 7 being a neutral solution, acidity increases below 7, alkalinity increases over 7.

POLYSORBATES   In this context, a group of agents used as emulsifiers in creams and lotions.

POLYVINYLPYRROLIDONE (PVP)   A water-soluble chemically inert substance used as a liquefacient in shampoo and hairspray and in emollient creams and rouge.

PRESERVATIVE   An agent added to a cosmetic to keep it stable and to prevent growth of contaminants.

PROPELLANT   A substance used to propel or spray the contents of an aerosol container.

PROPYLENE GLYCOL   A colorless viscous liquid used as an emulsifier, solvent, and wetting agent.

QUATERNARY AMMONIUM COMPOUNDS   Various compounds used in cosmetics as preservatives, germicides, and sanitizers.

RESIN   An insoluble thickener that contributes gloss and flow to certain cosmetics.

RESORCIN   A chemical compound derived from benzene used as an antiflaking agent in dandruff shampoos.

ROYAL JELLY   A nutritious secretion of a honeybee used as nectar for the queen bee and used by humans since ancient times for health and beauty.

SALICYLIC ACID A substance that acts as an antimicrobial agent in pharmaceuticals used to treat skin diseases.

SEQUESTERING AGENT An agent added to a cosmetic or other substance to prevent physical or chemical changes in the substance itself.

SHELLAC A type of lac from India derived from insect excretion and used in lacquer-type hairspray.

SODIUM BENZOATE A white, odorless powder used as a preservative and fungicide in bottled soda.

SODIUM LAURYL SULFATE A white or light yellow crystalline substance used in cosmetics as a detergent, wetting agent, and emulsifier.

SOLVENT A substance that can dissolve another substance.

SORBITOL A humectant used as a replacement for glycerin in emollients and nearly every other category of cosmetics.

SPERMACETI A wax obtained from the head of the sperm whale, used as an emollient and as a base for creams.

STEARIC ACID The most common fatty acid occurring in natural animal and vegetable salts and used in moisturizers and foundations as an emulsifier. The salts of stearic acid are called STEARATES.

STEROL A solid complex alcohol lubricant used as an emollient or emulsifier in many cosmetics.

SUNSCREEN An ingredient added to suntan preparations to filter out ultraviolet rays and prevent painful sunburn.

SURFACTANT An agent that reduces surface tension of liquids and is used in lotions to make them more spreadable and in creams to keep them from separating.

TALC A finely powdered mineral magnesium silicate that adds a slippery feeling to face and body powders, of which it is a component.

THICKENER A substance such as gum that adds body to lotions and creams.

TITANIUM DIOXIDE A white powdery substance used in lotions and cosmetic powders as a protectant. Also used in cosmetics as a pearling agent.

TONER A delicate lotion, similar to a freshener, used in cosmetics to make the skin feel tightened, refreshed, and cool.

ULTRAMARINE   An inorganic pigment used in eye cosmetics for shades of blue.

VANISHING CREAM   A surface cream used to soften the skin.

WITCH HAZEL   An alcoholic solution of an extract made from the leaves and bark of the witch hazel bush (*Hamamelis virginiana*), used on the skin as a mild local anesthetic and astringent.

ZINC OXIDE   A fine white powder used directly on the skin or in ointment as an astringent or healing agent and to remove the redness from skin blemishes. Also used as a pearling agent in cosmetics.